ONE POT **KETO**

Publications International, Ltd.

Pictured on the front cover: Chicken Scarpiello *(page 112)*.

Pictured on the back cover *(top to bottom):* Broccoli Cream Soup with Green Onions *(page 42)*, Forty-Clove Chicken Filice *(page 120)* and Steak Fajitas *(page 58)*.

Contributing Writer: Jacqueline B. Marcus, MS, RDN, LDN, CNS, FADA, FAND

ISBN: 978-1-64030-723-0

Manufactured in China.

8 7 6 5 4 3 2 1

Microwave Cooking: Microwave ovens vary in wattage. Use the cooking times as guidelines and check for doneness before adding more time.

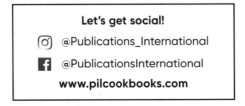

Let's get social!
@Publications_International
@PublicationsInternational
www.pilcookbooks.com

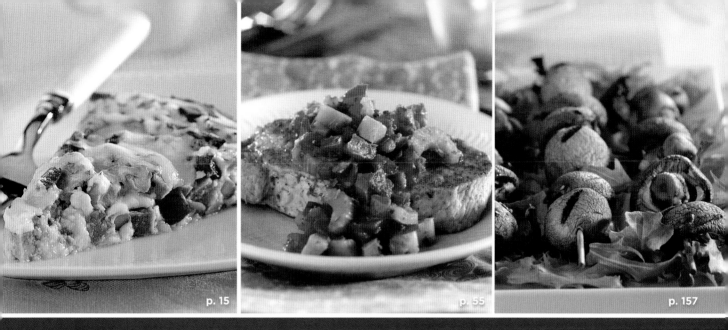

p. 15   p. 55   p. 157

CONTENTS

INTRODUCTION

DIETARY FATS AND OILS, WEIGHT AND HEALTH

Want to hear some good news about dietary fats and oils—especially how they relate to weight and health?

Consuming dietary fats and oils is not as bad as you might think—nor will consuming dietary fats and oils necessarily make you fat. The right amounts and types of dietary fats and oils may actually be satisfying and contribute to weight loss and weight maintenance. Dietary fats and oils are essential to your overall diet. Understanding what dietary fats and oils are and how they fit into an overall diet will help you with food selection, preparation and meal and menu planning.

The keto diet is based on ketones, organic compounds that are produced when dietary carbohydrates are limited. Ketosis is a normal metabolic process whereby the body burns stored fats instead of glucose from carbohydrates for energy. A diet based on ketosis, with its abundance of dietary fats and oils may actually help your dieting efforts. Understanding more about ketones and their place in a ketogenic diet may assist your food choices and dietary efforts.

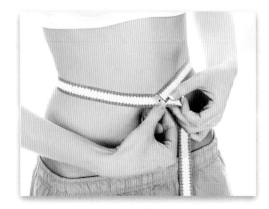

In addition to their role in weight loss and weight management, different types of dietary fats and oils and ketones are important for brain function, some disease protection and management, and overall health if used advantageously and correctly.

Dietary fats and oils are naturally found in foods and beverages such as dairy products, eggs, nuts, meats and seeds. Manufactured dietary fats and oils are found in some beverages, processed foods like margarine, cheeses and meats. Ketones are produced by the human body—you'll soon discover how.

There are differing viewpoints on the benefits of different types of dietary fats and oils and about ketones, the ideal amounts to consume and how ketones may sensibly be used for weight loss.

The purpose of this book is to help educate you about the types of dietary and blood fats and their contribution to health, and their relation to ketones and the ketogenic diet. It provides you with recipes that focus on healthy fats, proteins and non-starchy vegetables and de-emphasizes carbohydrates—particularly those that are refined or processed.

Your healthcare provider may help you determine if these approaches to eating and dieting are appropriate for you, so ask your doctor before you begin this or any other diet program.

CHOOSE THE RIGHT FATS

Fats are essential for proper body functioning and contribute satisfaction to diets, plus fats add flavor to foods and beverages. Still, fats provide more than twice the number of calories as carbohydrates or proteins (9 calories per gram compared to 4 calories per gram respectively). On a ketogenic diet, there is a different approach to fats than other diets that may restrict fats. The key is to understand the importance of fats in ketogenic diets and how to use them to your advantage.

> THE KEY IS TO UNDERSTAND THE IMPORTANCE OF FATS IN KETOGENIC DIETS AND HOW TO USE THEM TO YOUR ADVANTAGE.

TYPES OF FATS

Saturated fats are primarily found in foods from animal sources, such as meat, poultry and full-fat dairy products, while trans fats are mostly created when oils are partially hydrogenated to improve their cooking applications and to give them a longer shelf life. Saturated and trans fats may place a person at greater risk for heart disease. On the other hand, unsaturated fats that include monounsaturated and polyunsaturated fatty acids, found in plant-based foods such as avocados, nuts and seeds and olives and olive oil, and in fatty fish such as salmon, sardines and tuna tend to lower the risk of heart issues.

The American Heart Association (AHA) Diet and Lifestyle Recommendations suggest that a person limit saturated and trans fats and replace them with monounsaturated and polyunsaturated fats. If blood cholesterol needs to be lowered, then the recommendation is to reduce saturated fat to no more than 5 to 6 percent of total calories. For someone consuming 2,000 calories a day, this is about 13 grams of saturated fat, or about 117 calories. This is the equivalent of about 1 ounce of Cheddar cheese (9.4% total fat with 6 grams of saturated fat) and about 3 ounces of regular ground beef (25% total fat with 6.1 grams of saturated fat).

Try to eliminate trans fats (fats that have been processed into saturated fats) completely, or limit them to less than 1 percent of total daily calories. On a 2,000-calorie diet, this means that fewer than 20 calories (about 2 grams) should be derived from trans fats.

Table 1

KETOGENIC DIET BASICS

Generally, the percentages of macronutrients on a ketogenic diet are as follows:

- **Fat** 60 to 75 percent of total daily calories
- **Protein** 15 to 30 percent of total daily calories
- **Carbohydrates** 5 to 10 percent of total daily calories

Both fat and protein have high priority on a ketogenic diet, with non-starchy carbohydrates completing the remaining calories. While calories are not as important on the ketogenic diet as they are for other diets, a closer examination of the contributions of these macronutrients helps to put the amounts into perspective.

If total daily calories were about 2,000, then the percentages of macronutrients on a ketogenic diet would resemble the following amounts:

- **Fat** 60 to 75 percent of total daily calories or about 1,200 to 1,500 calories
- **Protein** 15 to 30 percent of total daily calories or about 300 to 600 calories
- **Carbohydrates** 5 to 10 percent of total daily calories or about 100 to 200 calories

In selecting foods and beverages, think protein and fat first, then non-starchy carbohydrates to complete. Until you truly have a handle on what constitutes low carbohydrates, find a carbohydrate counter to help to keep you in line. The ketogenic diet meal suggestions in Table 5 – SAMPLE KETOGENIC DIET MEALS: BREAKFAST, LUNCH, DINNER AND SNACKS on page 12 may help your food and beverage selections.

Table 2

ADVANTAGES AND DRAWBACKS OF KETOGENIC DIETS

ADVANTAGES	DRAWBACKS
• No calorie counting or focus on portion sizes	• Hard to sustain
• Initial weight loss	• Limited food choices
• After initial transition, hunger subsides	• May lead to taste fatigue
• Improved energy	• Socialization difficult
• Improved blood pressure	• Digestive issues (such as constipation, fatty stool, nausea)
• Improved blood fats: high-density lipoproteins, cholesterol, low-density lipoproteins, triglycerides	• Nutrient deficiencies (such as calcium, vitamins A, C and D, B-vitamins, fiber, magnesium, selenium)
• Reduced blood sugar, C-reactive protein (marker of inflammation), insulin, waist circumference	• Fiber, vitamin and mineral supplements suggested
• Significant short-term weight loss possible	• Increased urination (bladder, kidney contraindications)
	• Diabetes issues
	• Rapid, sizeable short-term weight loss concerning; long-term weight maintenance questionable

THE KETOGENIC DIET AND DIETING

The ketogenic diet is hardly new. The idea that fasting could be used as a therapy to treat disease was one that ancient Greek and Indian physicians embraced. "On the Sacred Disease," an early treatise in the Hippocratic Corpus, proposed how dietary modifications could be useful in epileptic management. Hippocrates, a Greek physician called the Father of Modern Medicine, wrote in "Epidemics" how abstinence from food and drink cured epilepsy.

In the 20th century, the first ketogenic diet became popularized in the 1920's and 30's as a regimen for treating epilepsy and an alternative to non-mainstream fasting. It was also promoted as a means of restoring health. In 1921, the ketogenic diet was officially established when an endocrinologist noted that three water-soluble compounds were produced by the liver as a result of following a diet that was rich in fat and low in carbohydrates. The term "water diet" had been used prior to this time to describe a diet that was free of starch and sugar. This is because when carbohydrates are broken down by the body carbon dioxide and water are by-products. When newer, anticonvulsant therapies were established, the ketogenic diet was temporarily abandoned.

In the 1960's the ketogenic diet was revisited when it was noted that more ketones are produced by medium chain triglycerides (MCTs) per unit of energy than by normal dietary fats (mostly long-chain triglycerides) because MCTs are quickly transported to the liver to be metabolized. In research diets where about 60 percent of the calories came from MCT oil, more protein and up to about three times as many carbohydrates could be consumed in comparison to "classic" ketogenic diets. This is why MCT oil is included in some ketogenic diets today.

In the 1950's and 1960's many versions of the ketogenic diet were popularized as high-protein, low-carbohydrate and a quick method of weight loss. Also at this time, the risk factors of excess fat and protein in the diet were criticized for being detrimental to health. Outside of the medical community, the ketogenic diet was not widely recognized for its therapeutic benefits so response to it was sensational in scope.

Then in the 1980's the Glycemic Index (GI) of foods and beverages was revealed that accounted for the differences in the speed of digestion of different types of carbohydrates. This explanation became the springboard for a number of ketogenic diets that were revised from years earlier. By the late 1990's the low-carb craze became one of the most popular types of dieting. Since this time, the original ketogenic diet underwent many refinements and hybrid diets developed.

Variations of the ketogenic diet continued to surface throughout the 20th century since the premise of the ketogenic diet—higher fat and protein and low carbohydrate—was used to treat diabetes and induce weight loss among other applications.

Table 1 summarizes the ketogenic diet basics. Many clinical studies examined their effectiveness and safety and their advantages and drawbacks were identified. These are condensed in **Table 2**.

FAT IN HEALTH AND DISEASE

Fats are essential to the diet and health for many purposes. Fats function as the body's thermostat. The layer of fat just beneath the skin helps to keep the body warm or causes it to perspire to cool the body.

Fat contributes to bile acids, cell membranes and steroid hormones (such as estrogen and testosterone), cushions the body from shock and helps to regulate fluid balance. Too many or too few fats in the diet may influence each of these important body functions.

One of the most important roles of fat in the body is as an energy source, especially when carbohydrates are not available from the diet or are lacking in the body. When people did manual work all day and expended the calories that they consumed, they made good use of carbohydrates and fats in their diet and within their energy stores. Today's laborsaving devices and sedentary lifestyles create less need for excess carbohydrate calories—particularly if they are refined. Even a plant-based diet may be unnecessarily high in refined carbohydrate calories.

Over the years, as humans moved from a plant-based diet toward an animal-based diet, the composition of fatty acids in the American diet switched from monounsaturated and polyunsaturated fats to more saturated fats, which are associated more with cardiovascular disease. A diet that is only filled with saturated fats may not be healthy. Incorporating avocado, fish, nuts, oils and seeds and other foods that contain monounsaturated and polyunsaturated fats into your diet may help to support a healthier proportion of fats in the body for weight maintenance and good health.

Besides cardiovascular disease, excess saturated and trans fats in the human diet are associated with certain cancers, cerebral vascular disease, diabetes, obesity and metabolic syndrome (a collection of conditions that may include abnormal cholesterol or triglyceride levels, excess body fat around the waist, high blood sugar and increased blood pressure that may increase a person's risk of diabetes, heart disease and/or stroke).

THE CHOLESTEROL CONTROVERSY

Atherosclerosis, or hardening of the arteries, is not a modern disease. Rather, the association between blood cholesterol and cardiovascular disease was recognized as far back as the 1850's.

One hundred years later in the 1950's, cholesterol and saturated fats in the diet were implicated as major risk factors for cardiovascular disease. Then in the 1980's, major US health institutions established that the process of lowering blood cholesterol (specifically LDL-cholesterol) reduces the risk of heart attacks that are caused by coronary heart disease.

Some scientists questioned this conclusion that marked the unofficial start of what's been called the "cholesterol controversy." Studies of cholesterol-lowering drugs known as statins supported the idea that reducing blood cholesterol means less mortality from heart disease. Subsequent statin studies have questioned this association. Other factors aside from dietary cholesterol have since been identified that may lead to elevated blood cholesterol, such as trans fats.

The liver manufactures cholesterol, so reducing cholesterol in the diet should help to reduce blood cholesterol, coronary heart disease and the risk of heart attack. But in some individuals, the liver produces more cholesterol than the body requires and cardiovascular disease may still develop. Accordingly, dietary cholesterol does not necessarily predict cardiovascular disease or a heart attack.

> WHAT YOU'LL LIKELY END UP WITH IS A SATISFYING EATING PLAN WITH AMPLE PROTEIN, HEALTHY FATS AND MINIMAL CARBOHYDRATES THAT MAY HELP YOU TO FEEL FULL AND LOSE WEIGHT IN THE PROCESS.

While dietary cholesterol may be a measure for greater cardiovascular risks, cardiovascular disease and heart attacks are also dependent upon such lifestyle and genetic factors as age, diet, exercise, gender, genetics, medication and stress. Reducing hydrogenated fats, saturated fats and trans fats; incorporating mono- and polyunsaturated fats and losing weight to help better manage blood fats are other sensible measures to take.

Longer-term weight management is also a preventative measure in cardiovascular disease. Reducing cholesterol and saturated fat in the diet while integrating foods and beverages with mono- and polyunsaturated fats and oils, dietary fiber, antioxidants and other phytonutrients may lead to a decrease in overall calorie consumption and weight loss and an improvement in overall health.

SO WHAT (AND HOW) SHOULD I EAT?

If you want to lose body fat, then the general consensus is that you need to take in fewer calories than you burn for energy. For example, if you're an average woman over 40, decreasing your caloric intake may be a reasonable starting point. If you are of shorter stature and/or very inactive, or you haven't dropped any pounds after a few weeks, you may consider lowering your daily intake of calories by 100-calorie increments until you start seeing weight loss. But don't go much below 1,000 calories without your health care provider's supervision. (And be sure to check with your health care provider before making any major changes to your diet or activity level, especially if you have any serious health problems.)

Another approach to weight loss is the ketogenic diet that does not focus on calories. Instead, the ketogenic diet focuses on the composition of calories from fats, proteins and carbohydrates.

Table 3

ACCEPTABLE FOODS, BEVERAGES AND INGREDIENTS FOR KETOGENIC DIETS

BEVERAGES

- Broth
- Hard liquor
- Nut milks
- Unsweetened coffee, tea
- Water

EGGS

- Egg whites
- Powdered eggs
- Whole eggs

FATS AND OILS

- Butter
- Cocoa butter
- Coconut butter, cream and oil
- Ghee
- Lard
- Oils: avocado oil, macadamia nut oil, MCT oil, olive oil and cold-pressed vegetable oils (flax, safflower, soybean)
- Mayonnaise

FISH AND SEAFOOD

- Anchovies
- Fish (catfish, cod, flounder, halibut, mackerel, mahi-mahi, salmon, snapper, trout, tuna)
- Shellfish (clams, crab, lobster, mussels, oysters, scallops, squid)

FRUITS AND VEGETABLES

- Avocados
- Cruciferous vegetables (broccoli, brussels sprouts, cabbage, cauliflower, kohlrabi)
- Fermented vegetables (kimchi, sauerkraut)
- Leafy greens (bok choy, chard, endive, lettuce, kale, radicchio, spinach, watercress)
- Lemon and lime juice and peel
- Mushrooms
- Non-starchy vegetables (asparagus, bamboo shoots, celery, cucumber)
- Seaweed and kelp
- Squash (spaghetti squash, yellow squash, zucchini)
- Tomatoes (used in moderation in some keto diets)

DAIRY PRODUCTS

- Crème fraîche
- Greek yogurt
- Hard cheese (aged Cheddar, feta, Parmesan, Swiss)
- Heavy cream
- Soft cheese (Brie, blue, Colby, Monterey Jack, mozzarella)
- Sour cream
- Spreadable cheese (cream cheese, cottage cheese and mascarpone)

MEATS AND POULTRY

- Beef (ground beef, roasts, steak, stew meat)
- Goat (leg, loin, rack, saddle, shoulder)
- Lamb (leg, loin, rack, ribs, shank, shoulder)
- Organ meats (heart, kidneys, liver, tongue)
- Poultry with skin (such as chicken, duck, pheasant, quail, turkey)
- Pork (bacon and sausage without fillers, ground pork, ham, pork chops, pork loin, tenderloin)
- Tofu used in moderation in some keto diets)
- Veal (double, flank, leg, rib, shoulder, sirloin)

NON-DAIRY BEVERAGES

- Almond milk
- Cashew milk
- Coconut milk
- Soymilk (used in moderation in some keto diets)

NUTS AND SEEDS

- Nut butters (almond, macadamia)
- Seeds (chia, flax, poppy, sesame, sunflower)
- Whole nuts (almonds, Brazil nuts, macadamia, pecans, hazelnuts, pine nuts, walnuts)

PANTRY ITEMS

- Herbs (dried or fresh such as basil, cilantro, oregano, parsley, rosemary and thyme)
- Horseradish
- Hot sauce
- Mustard
- Pepper
- Pesto sauce
- Pickles
- Salad dressings (without sweeteners)
- Salt
- Spices (such as ground red pepper, chili powder, cinnamon and cumin)
- Unsweetened gelatin
- Vinegar
- Whey protein (unsweetened)
- Worcestershire sauce

Table 4

UNACCEPTABLE FOODS, BEVERAGES AND INGREDIENTS FOR KETOGENIC DIETS

- Alcohol other than hard liquor (beer, sugary alcoholic beverages, wine)
- Beans
- Breads and breadstuffs
- Cakes and pastries
- Candy
- Cereals
- Cookies
- Crackers
- Flours
- Fruit, all (fresh, dried)
- Grains (amaranth, barley, buckwheat, bulgur, corn, millet, oats, rice, rye, sorghum, sprouted grains, wheat)
- Legumes (lentils, peas)
- Margarines with trans fats
- Milk (full-fat milk is acceptable in some ketogenic diets)
- Oats and muesli
- Potatoes, all kinds (white, yellow, sweet)
- Quinoa
- Pasta
- Pizza
- Processed and refined snack foods
- Rice
- Root vegetables
- Soda
- Sports drinks
- Sugar and honey
- Syrup
- Wheat gluten
- Yams

Fats are satisfying because they take longer for the body to digest, and some are converted into ketones for energy. You don't want to skimp on proteins because protein helps maintain and build calorie-burning muscle and also keeps you satiated between meals. Choose protein sources that supply monounsaturated fats and other heart-healthy unsaturated fats; good options include fish, seafood, nuts and seeds. (Fatty fish, such as herring, mackerel, salmon and tuna contain polyunsaturated fats—especially disease-fighting omega-3 fatty acids). You'll need to replace highly processed and refined foods that are full of saturated and trans fats, sugar and refined carbohydrates with minimally processed fiber- and nutrient-rich foods that include non-starchy vegetables.

What you'll likely end up with is a satisfying eating plan with ample protein, healthy fats and minimal carbohydrates that may help you to feel full and lose weight in the process. It's also a plan that may help you to maintain weight loss over time in a modified manner.

If you've ever tried to lose weight before, you know how quickly between-meal hunger may sabotage your best efforts. When your stomach starts rumbling hours before your next meal, it's tempting to grab whatever is available. Often, that "whatever" is some unhealthy packaged snack food or beverage that is loaded with empty calories, sodium, sugars and/or unhealthy fats. Or, if you manage to ignore this hunger, you may become so ravenous at the next meal that you consume far more calories than your body actually needs.

To prevent hunger from spoiling your weight-loss efforts, eat when you are hungry and stop eating when you are full, whether a meal or snack. Try to consume meals and snacks that include a source of hunger-fighting protein and healthy fat, and count your carbs so as not to exceed the daily limit of 20 to 50 grams of non-starchy carbohydrates.

Table 5

SAMPLE KETOGENIC DIET MEALS: BREAKFAST, LUNCH, DINNER AND SNACKS

Examples of combinations of protein, low-carb, non-starchy vegetables and fats:

BREAKFAST:

- Almond, coconut, hemp or other nut or seed milks or beverages (unsweetened)
- Bacon, sausage or sliced meats (without carbohydrate fillers)
- Cheese, hard or soft varieties
- Eggs, scrambled or fried + vegetables (asparagus, broccoli, garlic, mushrooms, onions or spinach) + coconut or olive oil + avocado, olives, salsa and/or sour cream
- Greek yogurt with nut butter, chia or flax seeds, herbs and spices (cinnamon, ginger or nutmeg)
- Smoked fish (such as lox, sable or whitefish)
- Smoothies made with keto-friendly ingredients (protein powder, almond or coconut butter, avocado, cocoa powder, chia or flax seeds, spices such as cinnamon, smoked paprika or turmeric and unsweetened almond or hemp milk)
- Vegetable slices (cucumber or zucchini or lettuce) topped with cheese

LUNCH AND DINNER:

- Eggs + watercress or spinach + avocado dressing
- Lamb + kale + sesame oil
- Pork + cauliflower + coconut butter
- Poultry + zucchini and yellow squash + extra virgin olive oil
- Salmon + broccoli + mustard sauce
- Sardines + cucumbers and onions + sour cream dressing
- Seafood + leafy green salad + oil and vinegar dressing
- Steak + asparagus + butter sauce
- Tofu + mushrooms and bok choy + ghee
- Tuna + celery + mayonnaise

SNACKS:

- Asparagus with goat cheese dip
- Avocado filled hard-cooked eggs
- Celery + nut or seed butter
- Cheese + olive skewers
- Chia and flaxseed crackers + cream cheese
- Cucumber and cream cheese spread
- Cream cheese and bacon stuffed celery
- Deviled eggs with fresh herbs and chives
- Greek yogurt with chopped cucumbers and garlic
- Guacamole with onions and garlic
- Ham and Cheddar or Swiss cheese roll ups
- Mixed nut-coated cheese balls
- Nut butters (such as almond) blended with ricotta cheese
- Olives stuffed with blue cheese
- Parmesan cheese crisps
- Seeds and seed butters such as tahini
- Sliced jicama with herbed cream cheese

Drink plenty of water throughout the day (especially if you live in a hot climate or sweat excessively) since ketogenic diets tend to be dehydrating and may lead to fatigue or ill feelings. This may be due to an imbalance of electrolytes; specifically sodium that the kidneys excrete during ketosis. Sometimes lightly salting your food may help to restore sodium. A high-quality vitamin and mineral supplement is also sensible.

NOTES ON KETOGENIC FOODS, BEVERAGES AND INGREDIENTS

In general, the foods, beverages and ingredients that are included in a ketogenic diet incorporate eggs, healthy fats and oils, fish, meats and organ meats and non-starchy vegetables. These "acceptable" foods, beverages and ingredients contain protein and fats and are low in carbohydrates that contribute to the effectiveness of ketogenic diets. They are listed in **Table 3 – ACCEPTABLE FOODS, BEVERAGES AND INGREDIENTS FOR KETOGENIC DIETS**.

In **Table 4 – UNACCEPTABLE FOODS, BEVERAGES AND INGREDIENTS FOR KETOGENIC DIETS** are shown. While there is a wide-range of ketogenic diet approaches, these foods, beverages and ingredients are generally considered to be "unacceptable" on many ketogenic diets. In general, their carbohydrate content exceeds what is considered as optimal for effective ketosis and diet success.

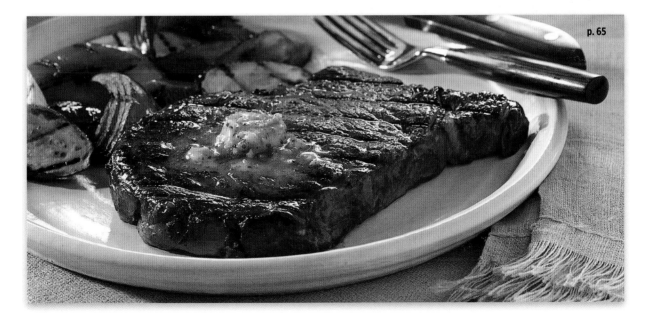

p. 65

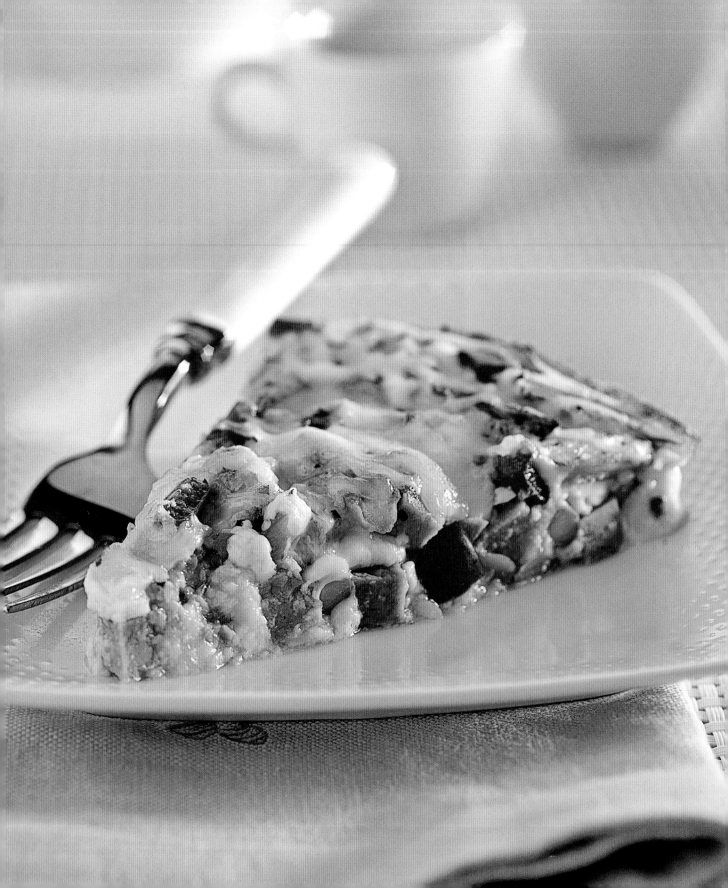

BREAKFAST

CRUSTLESS HAM AND ASPARAGUS QUICHE

- 2 cups sliced asparagus (½-inch pieces)
- 1 red bell pepper, chopped
- 1 tablespoon water
- 1 cup whole milk
- 4 eggs
- 4 ounces chopped cooked deli ham
- 2 tablespoons chopped fresh tarragon or basil
- ½ teaspoon salt
- ¼ teaspoon black pepper
- ½ cup (2 ounces) finely shredded Swiss cheese

1 Preheat oven to 350°F. Combine asparagus, bell pepper and water in microwavable bowl. Cover with waxed paper; microwave on HIGH 2 minutes or until vegetables are crisp-tender. Drain vegetables.

2 Whisk milk, egg whites and egg in large bowl until well blended. Stir in vegetables, ham, tarragon, salt and black pepper. Pour into 9-inch pie plate.

3 Bake 35 minutes. Sprinkle cheese over quiche; bake 5 minutes or until center is set and cheese is melted. Let stand 5 minutes before serving. Cut into 6 wedges.

MAKES 6 SERVINGS

PER SERVING

CALORIES 180, TOTAL FAT 10g, CARBS 7g, NET CARBS 5g, DIETARY FIBER 2g, PROTEIN 16g

ITALIAN SAUSAGE AND ARUGULA FRITTATA

1 tablespoon olive oil

2 links mild Italian turkey or pork sausage

2 tablespoons finely chopped red onion

12 cremini mushrooms, sliced

1 cup chopped arugula

¼ cup diced roasted red peppers

8 eggs

½ teaspoon salt

¼ teaspoon black pepper

¼ cup (1 ounce) shredded Italian cheese blend

1 Preheat oven to 350°F.

2 Heat oil in large ovenproof nonstick skillet over medium heat. Remove sausage from casings; add to skillet. Cook until almost browned, stirring to break up sausage. Add onion; cook and stir 1 minute or until softened. Add mushrooms; cook and stir 5 minutes. Stir in arugula and roasted peppers; cook and stir 1 minute or until heated through.

3 Whisk eggs, salt and black pepper in medium bowl until well blended. Pour over sausage mixture; sprinkle with cheese.

4 Bake 10 to 15 minutes or until center is set. Slide onto plate; cut into wedges. Serve warm or at room temperature.

MAKES 4 SERVINGS

VARIATION

For individual servings, spray 4 (6-ounce) ramekins or custard cups with nonstick cooking spray; place on baking sheet. Divide sausage and vegetable mixture evenly among prepared ramekins. Pour egg mixture over sausage mixture in each cup. Bake 25 to 30 minutes or until centers are set. Cool 10 minutes. (Frittatas will deflate slightly.)

PER SERVING

CALORIES 240, TOTAL FAT 18g, CARBS 4g, NET CARBS 3g, DIETARY FIBER 1g, PROTEIN 17g

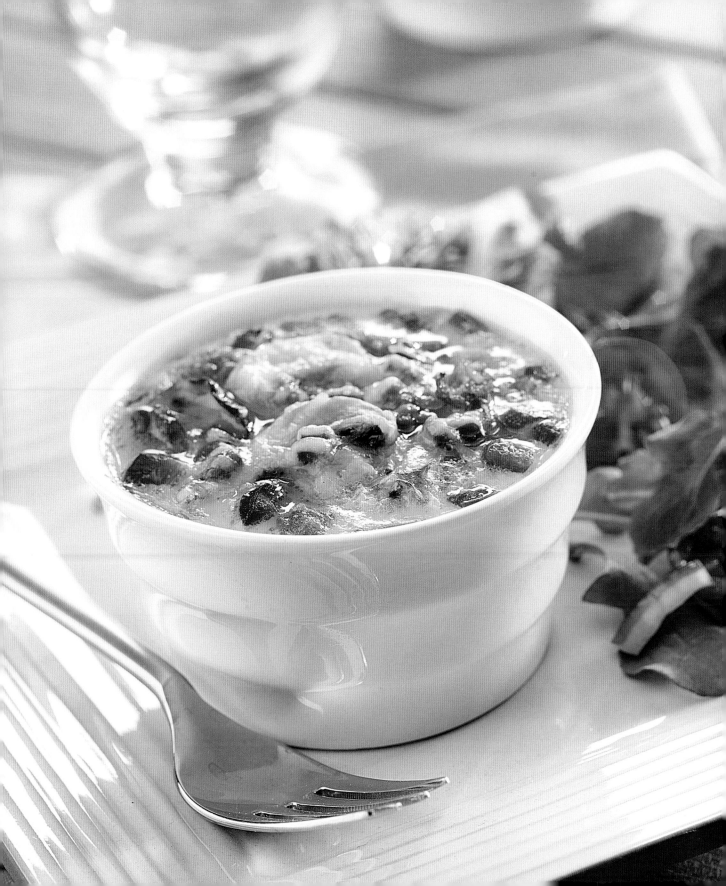

SAUSAGE AND CHEDDAR OMELET

2 uncooked turkey or pork breakfast sausage links (about 1 ounce each)

1 small onion, diced

Nonstick cooking spray *or* 2 teaspoons olive oil

1½ cups liquid egg substitute *or* 6 eggs, beaten

⅛ teaspoon salt

¼ teaspoon black pepper

½ cup (2 ounces) shredded Cheddar cheese, divided

Sliced green onions (optional)

1 Heat 12-inch nonstick skillet over medium-high heat. Remove sausage from casings. Add sausage and diced onion to skillet. Cook about 5 minutes or until sausage is no longer pink and onion is crisp-tender, stirring to break up meat. Transfer to bowl.

2 Wipe out skillet with paper towels; spray with cooking spray or place oil in skillet. Heat over medium-high heat. Pour egg substitute into skillet; sprinkle with salt and pepper. Cook 2 minutes or until bottom is set, lifting edge of egg to allow uncooked portion to flow underneath. Reduce heat to medium-low. Cover; cook 4 minutes or until top is set.

3 Gently slide cooked egg onto large serving plate; spoon sausage mixture down center. Sprinkle with ¼ cup cheese. Fold sides of omelet over sausage mixture. Sprinkle with remaining ¼ cup cheese and green onions, if desired. Cut into 4 pieces; serve immediately.

MAKES 4 SERVINGS

PER SERVING

CALORIES 133, TOTAL FAT 6g, CARBS 4g, NET CARBS 3g, DIETARY FIBER 1g, PROTEIN 15g

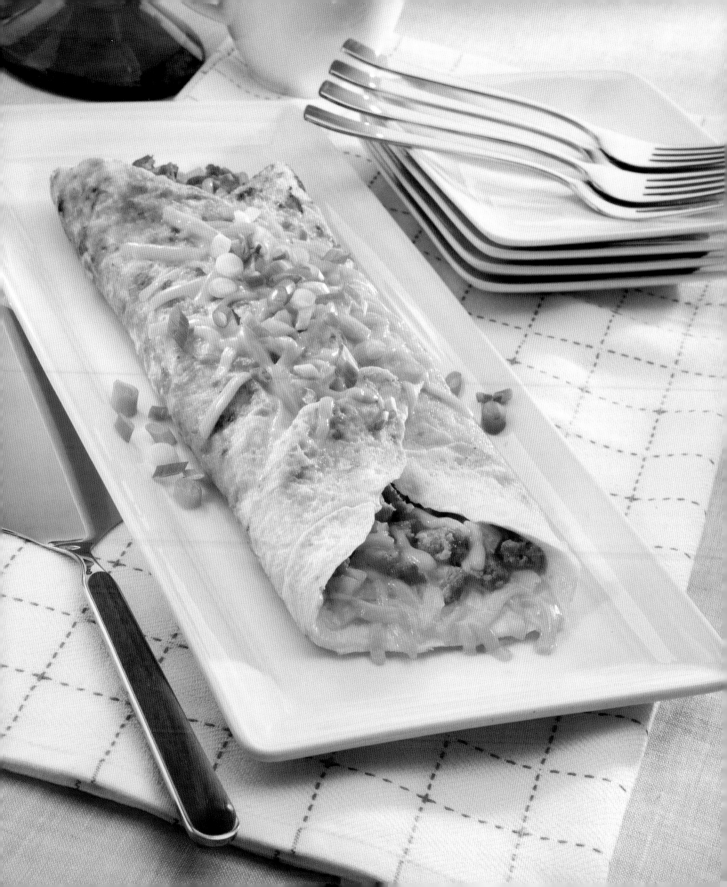

SPINACH AND HAM QUICHE

3 eggs

1 cup whole milk

¼ teaspoon salt

¼ teaspoon ground nutmeg

Pinch red pepper flakes

1 package (10 ounces) frozen chopped spinach, thawed and squeezed dry

1 cup (4 ounces) shredded mozzarella cheese

½ cup (about 2 ounces) chopped deli ham

⅓ cup chopped onion

1 clove garlic, minced

Salsa (optional)

1 Preheat oven to 350°F. Spray 8-inch square baking pan with nonstick cooking spray.

2 Whisk eggs, milk, salt, nutmeg and red pepper flakes in large bowl until well blended. Stir in spinach, cheese, ham, onion and garlic; mix well.

3 Pour into prepared baking pan. Bake about 40 minutes or until center is firm. Cut into 4 squares; serve with salsa, if desired.

MAKES 4 SERVINGS

PER SERVING

CALORIES 220, TOTAL FAT 13g, CARBS 8g, NET CARBS 6g, DIETARY FIBER 2g, PROTEIN 17g

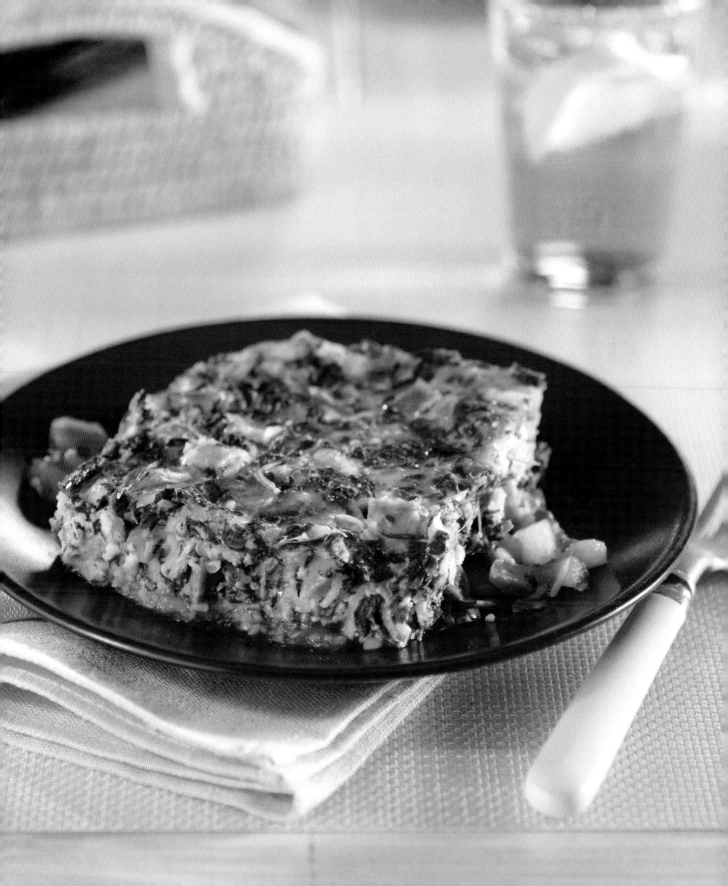

SPICY CRABMEAT FRITTATA

1 can (about 6 ounces) lump white crabmeat, drained

6 eggs

¼ teaspoon salt

¼ teaspoon black pepper

¼ teaspoon hot pepper sauce

1 tablespoon olive oil

1 green bell pepper, finely chopped

2 cloves garlic, minced

1 plum tomato, seeded and finely chopped

1 Preheat broiler. Pick out and discard any shell or cartilage from crabmeat; break up large pieces of crabmeat.

2 Whisk eggs in medium bowl. Add crabmeat, salt, black pepper and hot pepper sauce; mix well.

3 Heat oil in large ovenproof skillet over medium-high heat. Add bell pepper and garlic; cook and stir 3 minutes or until tender. Add tomato; cook and stir 1 minute. Stir in egg mixture; cook over medium-low heat 7 minutes or until eggs begin to set around edges.

4 Transfer skillet to broiler. Broil 4 inches from heat source 1 to 2 minutes or until frittata is golden brown and center is set.

MAKES 4 SERVINGS

PER SERVING

CALORIES 187, TOTAL FAT 11g, CARBS 4g, NET CARBS 3g, DIETARY FIBER 1g, PROTEIN 17g

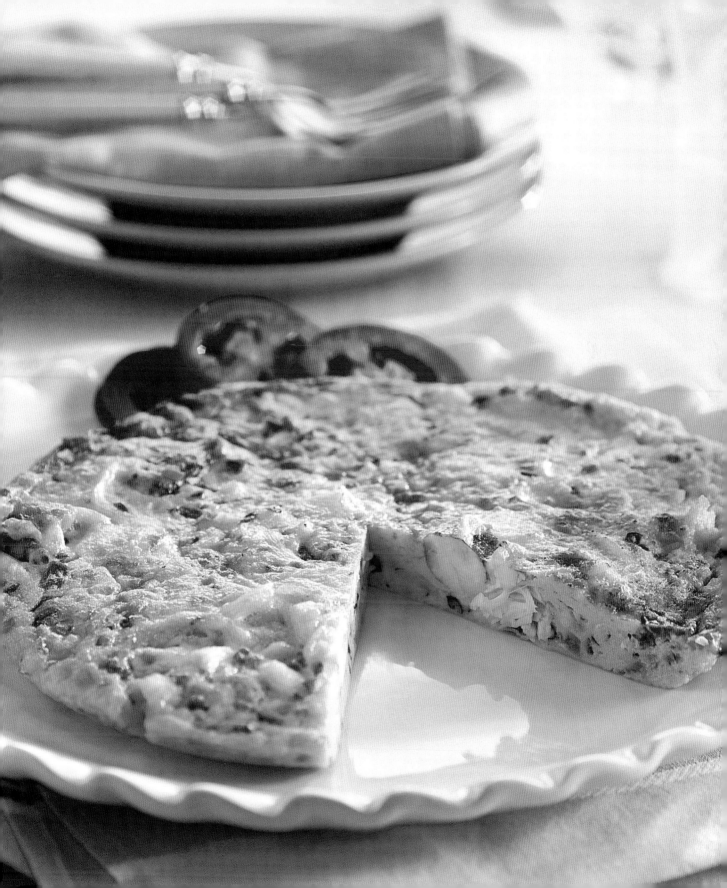

FETA BRUNCH BAKE

6 eggs

1 jarred roasted bell pepper, chopped

2 packages (10 ounces each) frozen chopped spinach, thawed and squeezed dry

1½ cups (6 ounces) crumbled feta cheese

⅓ cup chopped onion

2 tablespoons chopped fresh parsley

¼ teaspoon dried dill weed

Salt and black pepper

1 Preheat oven to 400°F. Spray 1-quart baking dish with nonstick cooking spray.

2 Whisk eggs in large bowl until foamy. Stir in roasted pepper, spinach, cheese, onion, parsley and dill weed; season with salt and black pepper. Pour into prepared baking dish.

3 Bake 20 minutes or until set. Let stand 5 minutes. Cut into 4 squares to serve.

MAKES 4 SERVINGS

PER SERVING

CALORIES 280, TOTAL FAT 18g, CARBS 10g, NET CARBS 6g, DIETARY FIBER 4g, PROTEIN 21g

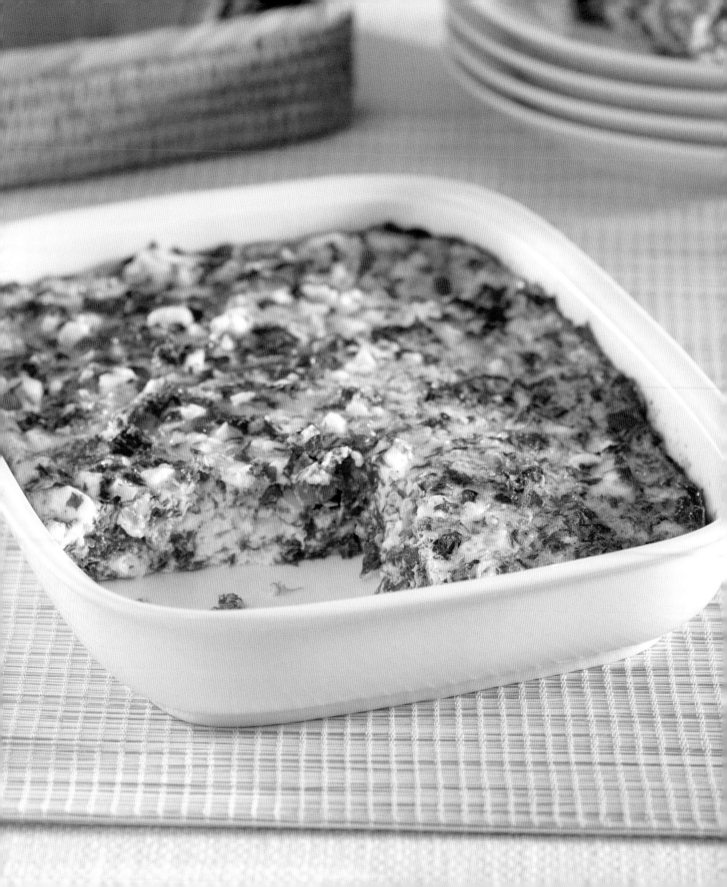

BROCCOLI AND HAM FRITTATA

3 eggs

3 egg whites

½ teaspoon salt

½ teaspoon black pepper

1½ cups (4 ounces) frozen broccoli florets, thawed

6 ounces smoked deli ham, cut into ½-inch cubes (1¼ cups)

⅓ cup jarred roasted red peppers, cut into thin strips

1 tablespoon butter

½ cup (2 ounces) shredded sharp Cheddar cheese

1 Preheat broiler.

2 Whisk eggs, egg whites, salt and black pepper in large bowl until blended. Stir in broccoli, ham and roasted peppers.

3 Melt butter in 10-inch ovenproof skillet over medium heat over medium-low heat. Pour egg mixture into skillet. Cover; cook 5 to 6 minutes or until eggs are set around edge. (Center will be wet.)

4 Uncover; sprinkle cheese over frittata. Transfer skillet to broiler. Broil 5 inches from heat 2 minutes or until center is set and cheese is melted. Let stand 5 minutes; cut into 4 wedges.

MAKES 4 SERVINGS

PER SERVING

CALORIES 211, TOTAL FAT 13g, CARBS 5g, NET CARBS 4g, DIETARY FIBER 1g, PROTEIN 19g

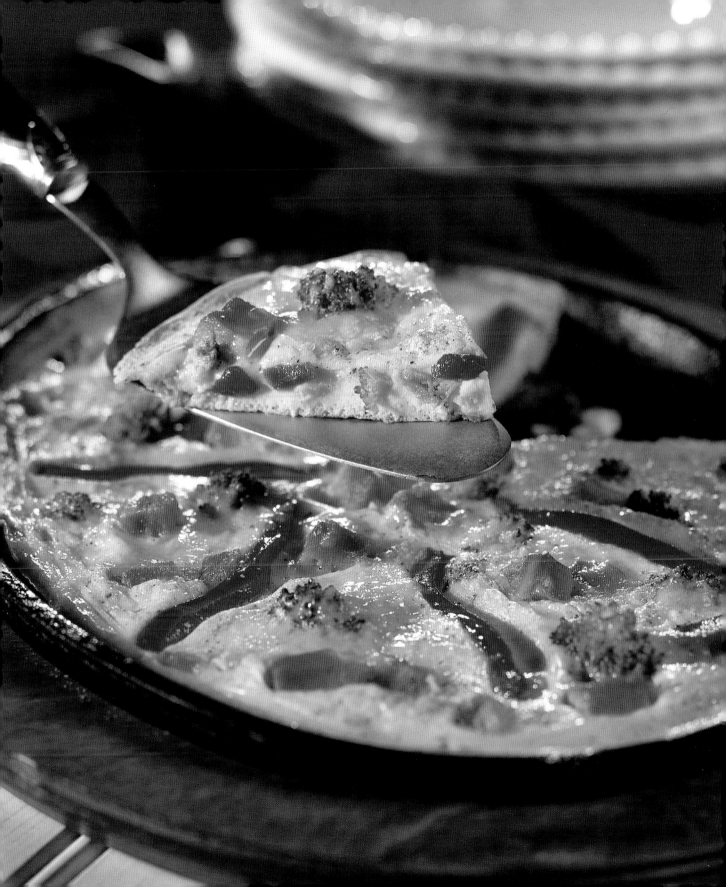

JOE'S SPECIAL

1 pound lean ground beef

2 cups sliced mushrooms

1 small onion, chopped

2 teaspoons Worcestershire sauce

1 teaspoon dried oregano

1 teaspoon ground nutmeg

½ teaspoon garlic powder

½ teaspoon salt

1 package (10 ounces) frozen chopped spinach, thawed

4 eggs, lightly beaten

⅓ cup grated Parmesan cheese

1 Spray large skillet with nonstick cooking spray; heat over medium-high heat. Add ground beef, mushrooms and onion; cook and stir 6 to 8 minutes or until meat is browned and vegetables are tender. Add Worcestershire sauce, oregano, nutmeg, garlic powder and salt.

2 Drain spinach (do not squeeze dry); stir into meat mixture. Push mixture to one side of skillet. Reduce heat to medium. Pour eggs into other side of skillet; cook without stirring 1 to 2 minutes or until set on bottom. Lift eggs to allow uncooked portion to flow underneath. Repeat until softly set. Gently stir into meat mixture and heat through. Stir in cheese.

MAKES 4 SERVINGS

PER SERVING

CALORIES 401, TOTAL FAT 25g, CARBS 9g, NET CARBS 6g, DIETARY FIBER 3g, PROTEIN 34g

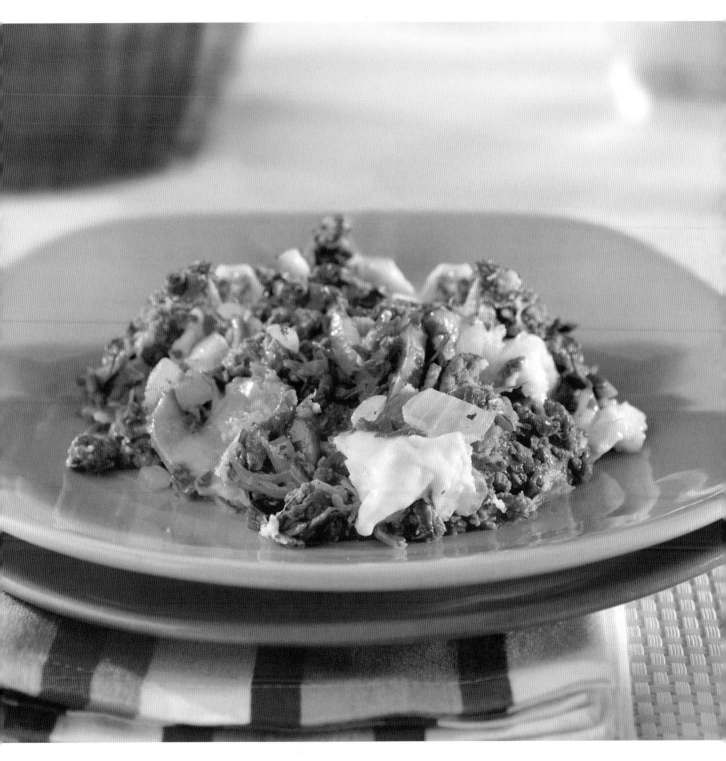

SPINACH, TOMATO AND CHEDDAR OMELET

1 package (5 ounces) fresh baby spinach

Nonstick cooking spray *or* 4 teaspoons olive oil

3 cups liquid egg substitute *or* 12 eggs, beaten, divided

2 plum tomatoes, diced (about ¾ cup)

1 cup (4 ounces) finely shredded extra-sharp Cheddar cheese

¼ teaspoon black pepper (optional)

1 Rinse spinach; drain, leaving water clinging to leaves. Place in small nonstick skillet. Cover and cook over medium-low heat until wilted. Transfer to bowl.

2 Wipe out skillet; spray with cooking spray or place 1 teaspoon oil in skillet; heat over medium heat. Pour ¾ cup egg substitute into skillet; cook about 2 minutes or until set, lifting edge to allow uncooked portion to flow underneath.

3 Spoon one fourth of spinach and one fourth of tomatoes over half of omelet; sprinkle with 2 tablespoons cheese and pepper, if desired. Fold opposite half of omelet over filling. Transfer to plate. Sprinkle with 2 tablespoons cheese. Repeat with remaining egg substitute, spinach, tomatoes and cheese to make 3 more omelets.

MAKES 4 SERVINGS

NOTE

To make just one omelet, use ½ cup packed baby spinach, ¾ cup egg substitute, 3 tablespoons diced tomato and ¼ cup cheese.

PER SERVING

CALORIES 222, TOTAL FAT 8g, CARBS 5g, NET CARBS 4g, DIETARY FIBER 1g, PROTEIN 31g

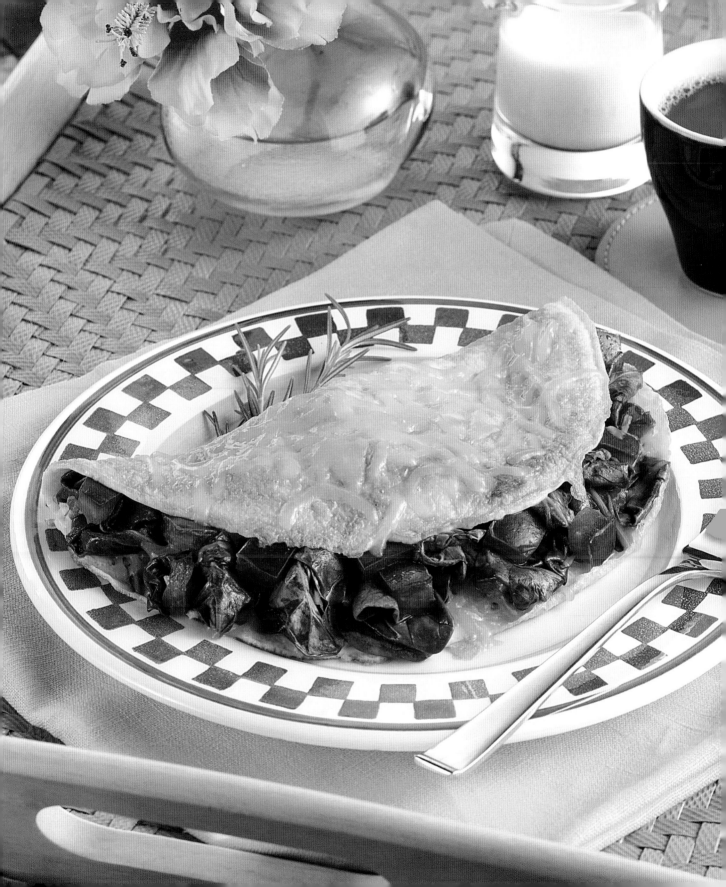

POBLANO SAUSAGE FRITTATA

4 eggs

¼ cup milk

1 package (12 ounces) bulk pork breakfast sausage

1 poblano pepper, seeded and chopped

1 cup (4 ounces) shredded Cheddar cheese

1 Preheat broiler. Whisk eggs and milk in medium bowl until well blended.

2 Heat 12-inch ovenproof nonstick skillet over medium-high heat. Add sausage; cook and stir 4 minutes or until no longer pink, stirring to break up meat. Transfer sausage to paper towels with slotted spoon. Drain fat.

3 Add pepper to same skillet; cook and stir 2 minutes or until crisp-tender. Return sausage to skillet. Add egg mixture; stir until blended. Cover; cook over medium-low heat 10 minutes or until eggs are almost set.

4 Sprinkle cheese over frittata; broil 2 minutes or until cheese is melted. Cut into 4 wedges. Serve immediately.

MAKES 4 SERVINGS

TIP

If your skillet is not ovenproof, wrap the handle in heavy-duty foil.

PER SERVING

CALORIES 423, TOTAL FAT 31g, CARBS 4g, NET CARBS 3g, DIETARY FIBER 1g, PROTEIN 27g

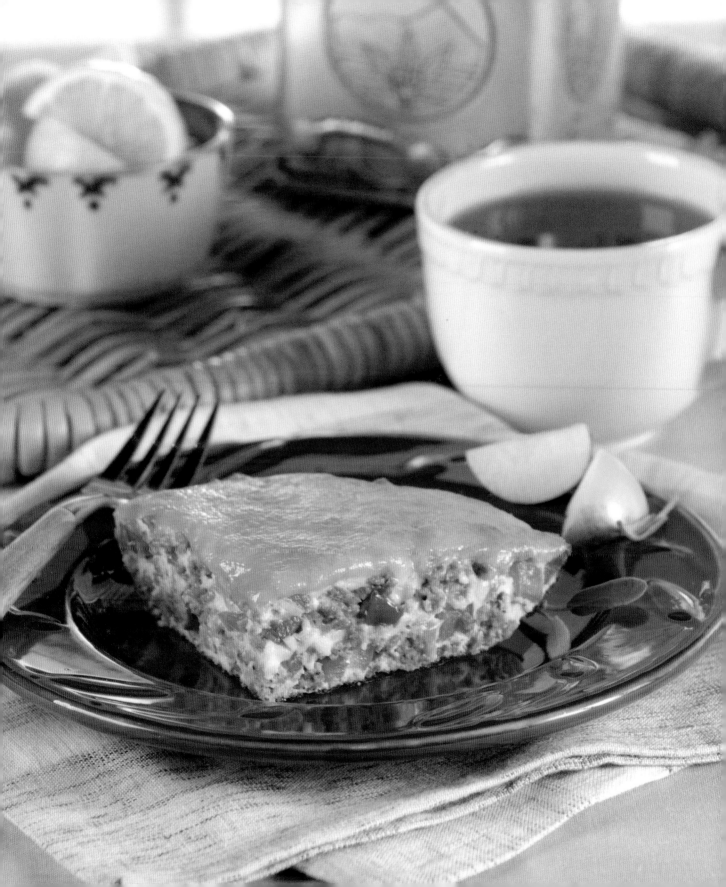

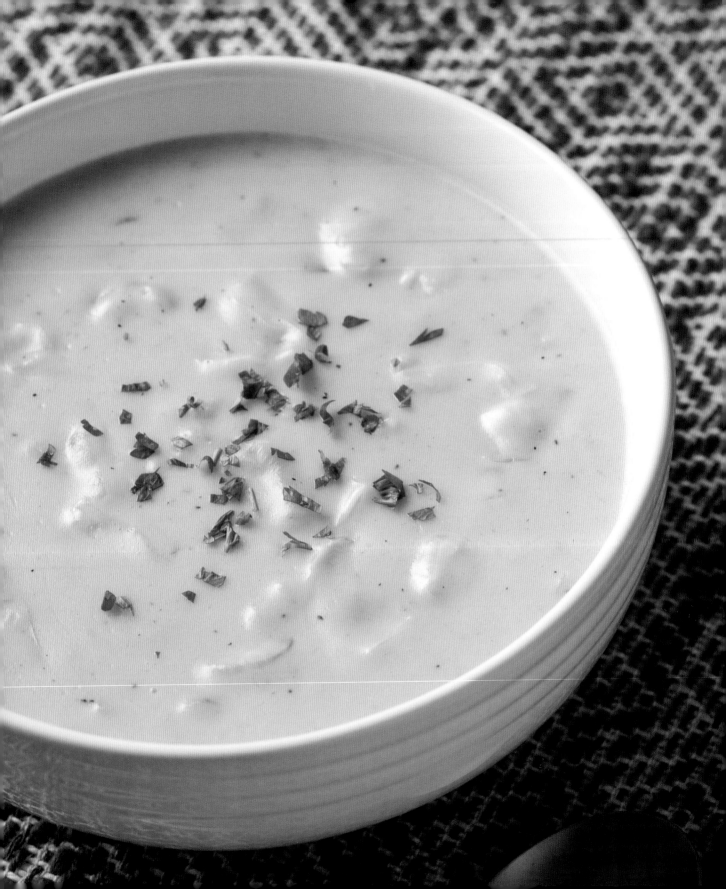

SOUPS & STEWS

CREAMY ONION SOUP

6 tablespoons
    (¾ stick) butter

1 large sweet onion,
    thinly sliced
    (about 3 cups)

1 can (about
    14 ounces) chicken
    broth

1½ cups milk

2 cubes chicken
    bouillon

¼ teaspoon black
    pepper

1½ cups (6 ounces)
    shredded Colby-
    Jack cheese

Chopped fresh
    parsley (optional)

1 Melt butter in large saucepan or Dutch oven over medium heat. Add onions; cook 10 minutes or until soft and translucent, stirring occasionally. Add broth, milk, bouillon and pepper; cook about 20 minutes until bouillon is dissolved and mixture is thickened slightly and hot but not boiling.

2 Add cheese; cook 5 minutes or until melted and smooth. Ladle into bowls; garnish with parsley.

MAKES 5 SERVINGS

PER SERVING

CALORIES 330, TOTAL FAT 26g, CARBS 10g,
NET CARBS 9g, DIETARY FIBER 1g, PROTEIN 10g

ASIAN FISH STEW

8 to 10 dried black Chinese mushrooms

¼ cup soy sauce

2 tablespoons Chinese rice wine

1 teaspoon chopped fresh ginger

Black pepper

8 ounces medium shrimp, peeled and deveined

8 ounces halibut, cubed

1 tablespoon vegetable oil

2 cloves garlic, chopped

2 cups diagonally sliced bok choy

1½ cups diagonally sliced napa cabbage

1 cup broccoli florets

2 cups vegetable broth

½ cup bottled clam juice or water

2 green onions with tops, sliced

1 Place mushrooms in medium bowl; cover with warm water. Soak 20 to 40 minutes or until soft. Cut off and discard stems; cut caps into thin slices. Set aside.

2 Whisk soy sauce, rice wine, ginger and pepper in small bowl until well blended. Add shrimp and halibut; marinate at room temperature 10 minutes.

3 Meanwhile, heat oil in Dutch oven or large saucepan over medium-high heat. Add garlic; cook and stir 3 to 5 minutes or until softened. Stir in bok choy, cabbage and broccoli.

4 Drain seafood, reserving marinade. Pour prepared vegetable broth, clam juice and reserved marinade into Dutch oven; bring to a boil over high heat. Reduce heat to low. Simmer 5 to 10 minutes until vegetables are crisp-tender. Add seafood and mushrooms. Simmer 3 to 5 minutes until shrimp are opaque and fish flakes easily when tested with fork.

MAKES 6 SERVINGS

PER SERVING

CALORIES 160, TOTAL FAT 4g, CARBS 12g, NET CARBS 9g, DIETARY FIBER 3g, PROTEIN 18g

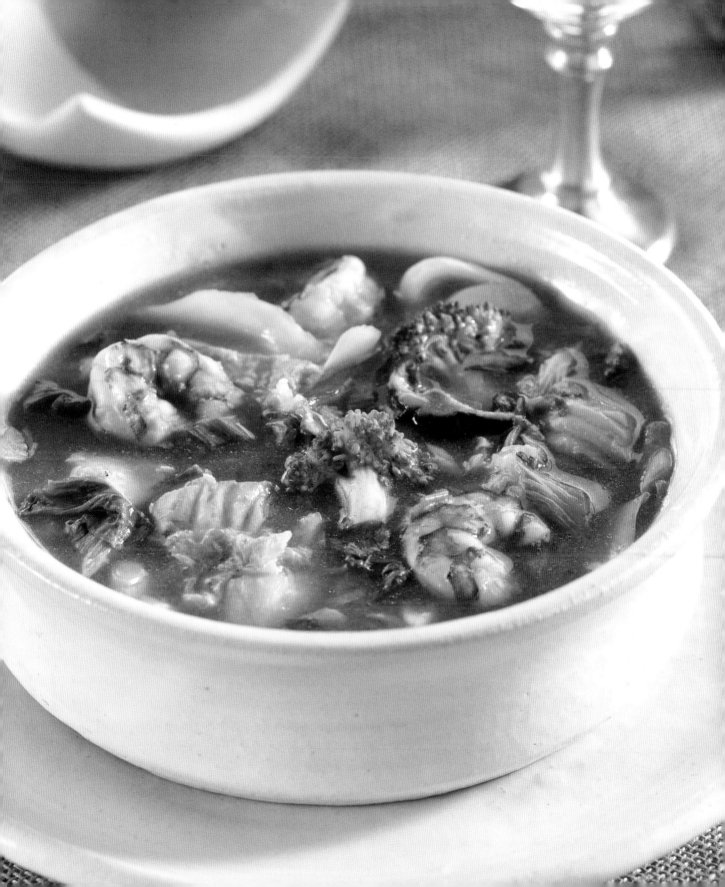

ROMAN SPINACH SOUP

6 cups chicken broth

1 cup liquid egg substitute

¼ cup minced fresh basil

3 tablespoons grated Parmesan cheese

2 tablespoons fresh lemon juice

1 tablespoon minced fresh parsley

¼ teaspoon white pepper

⅛ teaspoon ground nutmeg

8 cups packed fresh spinach, chopped

Fresh lemon slices (optional)

1 Bring broth to a boil in 4-quart saucepan over medium heat.

2 Whisk egg substitute, basil, Parmesan cheese, lemon juice, parsley, white pepper and nutmeg in small bowl. Set aside.

3 Stir spinach into broth; simmer 1 minute. Slowly pour egg mixture into broth mixture, whisking constantly so egg threads form. Simmer 2 to 3 minutes or until egg is cooked. Garnish with lemon slices. Serve immediately.

MAKES 8 SERVINGS

NOTE

Soup may look curdled.

PER SERVING

CALORIES 46, **TOTAL FAT** 1g, **CARBS** 4g, **NET CARBS** 3g, **DIETARY FIBER** 1g, **PROTEIN** 6g

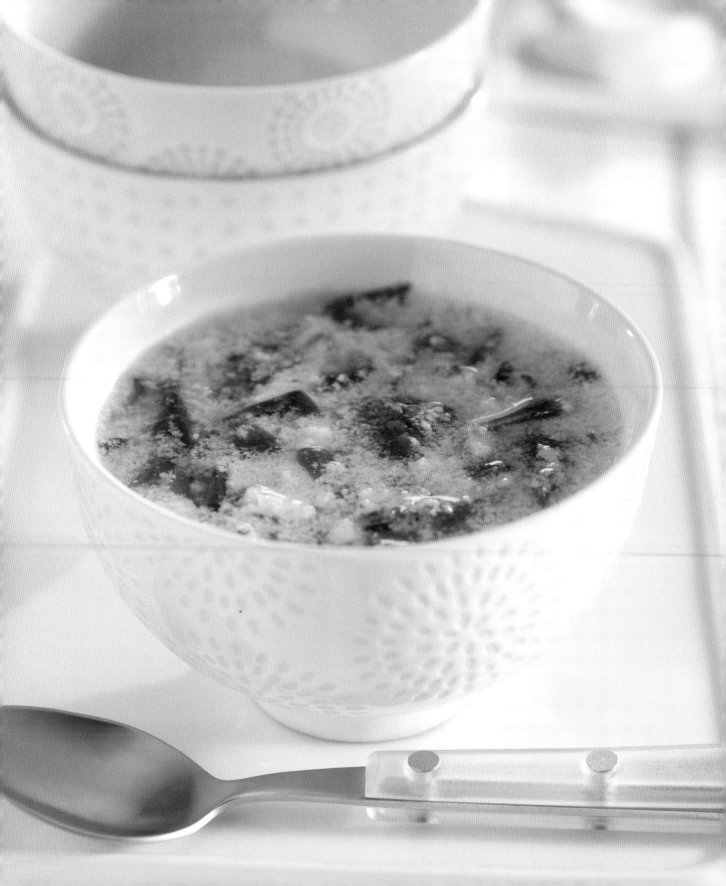

GREEK-STYLE KALE AND SAUSAGE STEW

1 tablespoon olive oil

1 small onion, diced

1 pound uncooked Portuguese or hot Italian sausage

6 cups (4 ounces) coarsely chopped kale leaves (trimmed of thick stems)

1¼ cups hot chicken broth, divided

2 eggs, beaten

3 tablespoons fresh lemon juice

1 Heat oil in large skillet over medium heat. Add onion; cook 5 minutes or until tender. Break sausage into bite-size pieces and add to skillet. Cook and stir 5 minutes or until sausage is browned on all sides. Stir in kale and ½ cup broth. Reduce heat to low; cover and simmer 20 minutes or until kale is tender.

2 Whisk eggs with lemon juice in medium bowl. Whisking constantly, add remaining ¾ cup hot broth in thin steady stream. Stir egg mixture into sausage mixture. Simmer over low heat 1 to 2 minutes or until egg mixture is slightly thickened. (Do not boil.)

MAKES 6 SERVINGS

PER SERVING

CALORIES 359, TOTAL FAT 26g, CARBS 11g, NET CARBS 9g, DIETARY FIBER 2g, PROTEIN 21g

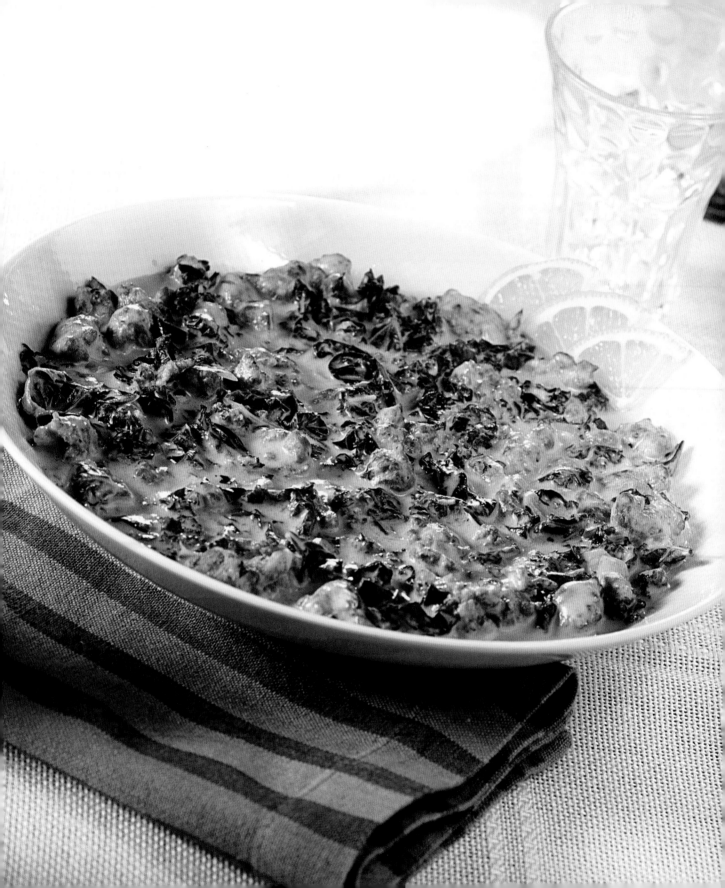

BROCCOLI CREAM SOUP

1 tablespoon olive oil

2 cups chopped onions

1 pound fresh or frozen broccoli florets or spears

2 cups chicken or vegetable broth

6 tablespoons cream cheese

1 cup milk

¾ teaspoon salt

⅛ teaspoon ground red pepper

Finely chopped green onions (optional)

1 Heat oil in large saucepan over medium-high heat. Add onions; cook and stir 4 minutes or until translucent. Add broccoli and broth; bring to a boil. Reduce heat to medium-low; cover and simmer 10 minutes or until broccoli is tender.

2 Working in batches, process mixture in food processor or blender until smooth. (Or use handheld immersion blender.) Return mixture to saucepan; heat over medium heat.

3 Whisk in cream cheese until melted. Stir in milk, salt and red pepper; cook 2 minutes or until heated through. Top with green onions, if desired.

MAKES 6 SERVINGS

PER SERVING

CALORIES 150, TOTAL FAT 10g, CARBS 13g, NET CARBS 10g, DIETARY FIBER 3g, PROTEIN 6g

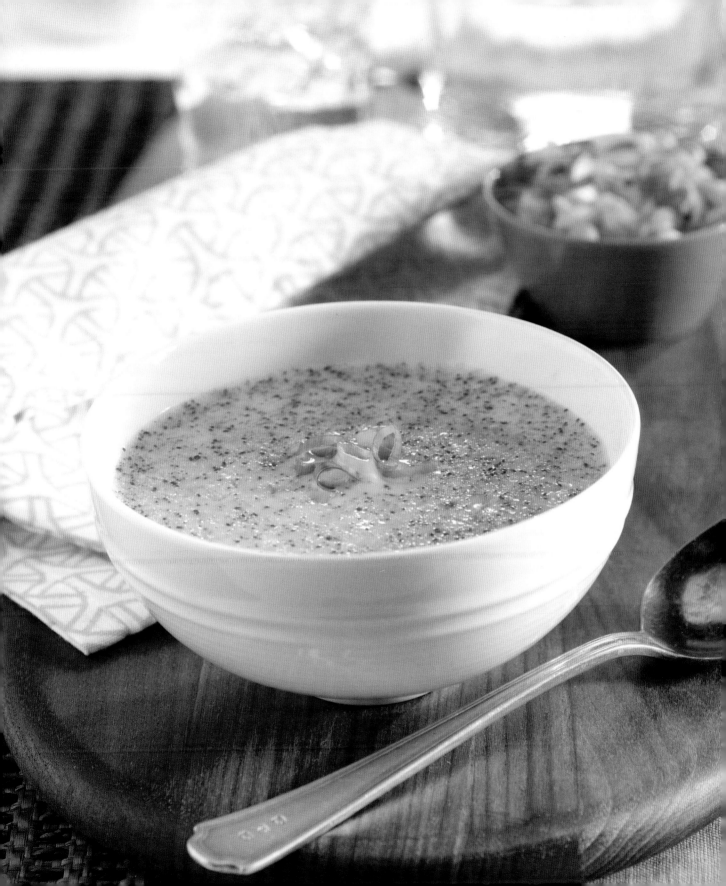

CHUNKY TOMATO-BASIL SOUP

2 tablespoons olive oil

1 cup chopped onion

2 cloves garlic, minced

5 cups fresh tomatoes, peeled, seeded and chopped, divided

1 can (6 ounces) tomato paste

1½ teaspoons dried basil

¼ teaspoon salt

½ teaspoon dried marjoram

¼ teaspoon black pepper

4 cups chicken or vegetable broth

1 Heat oil in large saucepan over medium heat. Add onion and garlic; cover and cook 7 minutes or until onion is tender, stirring occasionally.

2 Reserve 1 cup fresh tomatoes. Add remaining tomatoes to saucepan. Stir in tomato paste, basil, salt, marjoram and pepper. Stir in broth. Bring to a boil. Reduce heat; cover and simmer 30 minutes.

3 Pour about one third of hot soup into blender. Cover loosely and blend until smooth. Repeat with remaining soup, one third at a time. Return puréed soup to saucepan. (Or use handheld immersion blender.) Stir in reserved tomatoes. Cook until heated through.

MAKES 6 SERVINGS

PER SERVING

CALORIES 110, **TOTAL FAT** 5g, **CARBS** 13g, **NET CARBS** 10g, **DIETARY FIBER** 3g, **PROTEIN** 4g

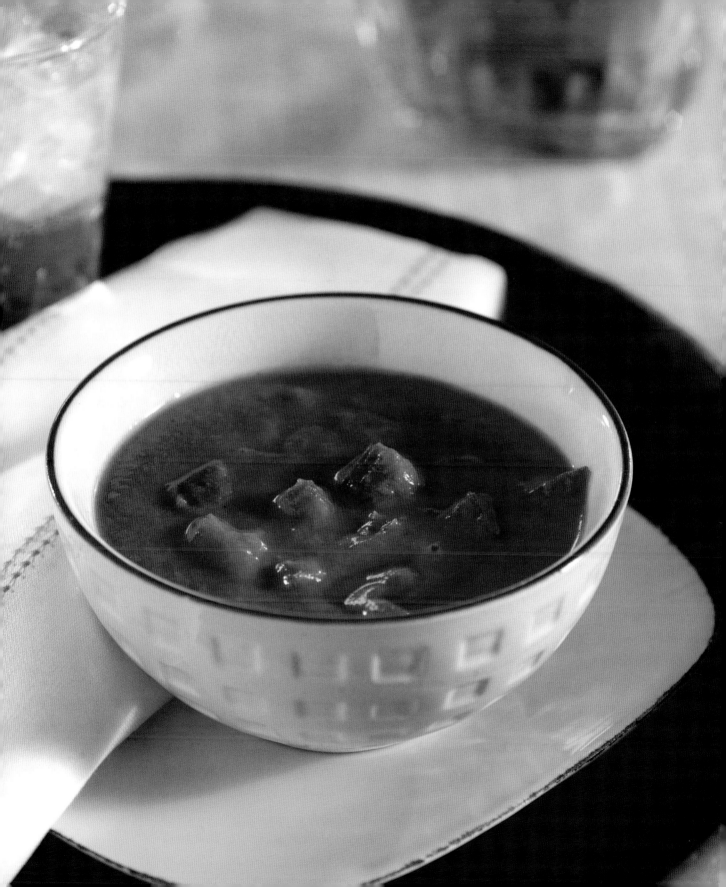

BEEFY BROCCOLI SOUP

4 ounces ground beef

2 cups beef broth

1 bag (10 ounces) frozen chopped broccoli, thawed

¼ cup chopped onion

1 cup milk

1 cup (4 ounces) shredded sharp Cheddar cheese

1½ teaspoons chopped fresh oregano *or* ½ teaspoon dried oregano

Salt and black pepper

Hot pepper sauce

1 Brown beef in large saucepan over medium-high heat 6 to 8 minutes, stirring to break up meat. Drain fat; transfer beef to bowl.

2 Bring broth to a boil in same saucepan over medium-high heat. Add broccoli and onion; cook 5 minutes or until broccoli is tender. Stir in milk and beef; cook and stir until mixture is thickened and heated through.

3 Add cheese and oregano; stir until cheese is melted. Season with salt, black pepper and hot pepper sauce.

MAKES 4 SERVINGS

PER SERVING

CALORIES 260, TOTAL FAT 16g, CARBS 8g, NET CARBS 6g DIETARY FIBER 2g, PROTEIN 19g

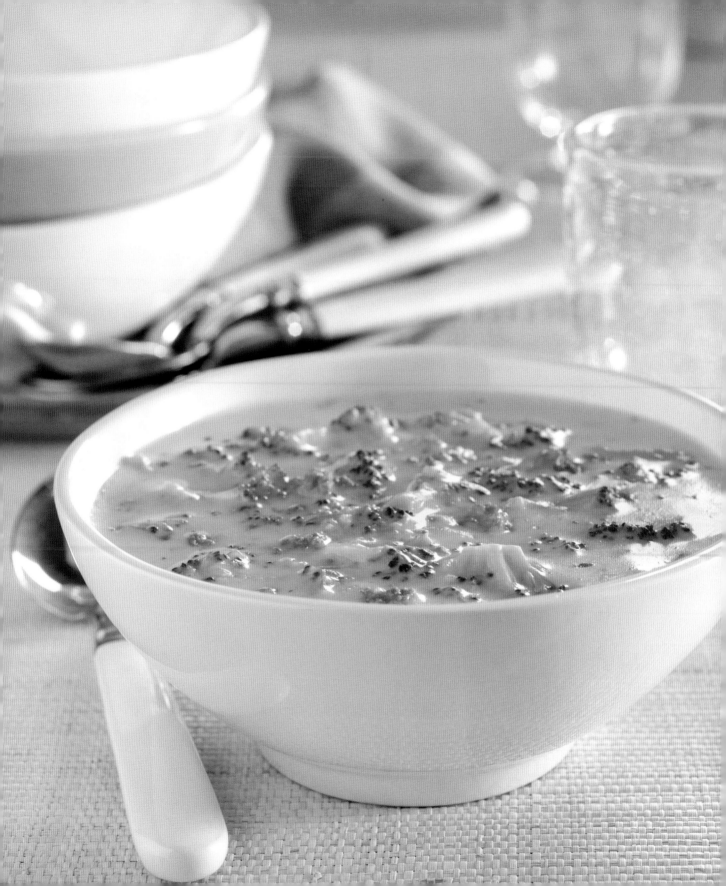

COLD YOGURT SOUP

1 cup finely chopped
   cooked chicken

1 teaspoon lemon juice

¾ teaspoon minced
   fresh *or* ¼ teaspoon
   dried dill weed

½ teaspoon salt

⅛ teaspoon garlic
   powder

   Pinch white pepper

2 cups plain whole milk
   yogurt

1 small cucumber,
   seeded and diced

⅓ cup chopped celery

3 tablespoons thinly
   sliced green onions

   Thin radish slices
   (optional)

1 Place chicken, lemon juice, dill, salt, garlic powder and pepper in large bowl; toss lightly. Cover and refrigerate 30 minutes.

2 Stir in yogurt, cucumber, celery and green onion. Pour soup into serving bowls; garnish with radish slices.

MAKES 4 SERVINGS

PER SERVING

CALORIES 150, TOTAL FAT 6g, CARBS 10g, NET CARBS 9g, DIETARY FIBER 1g, PROTEIN 13g

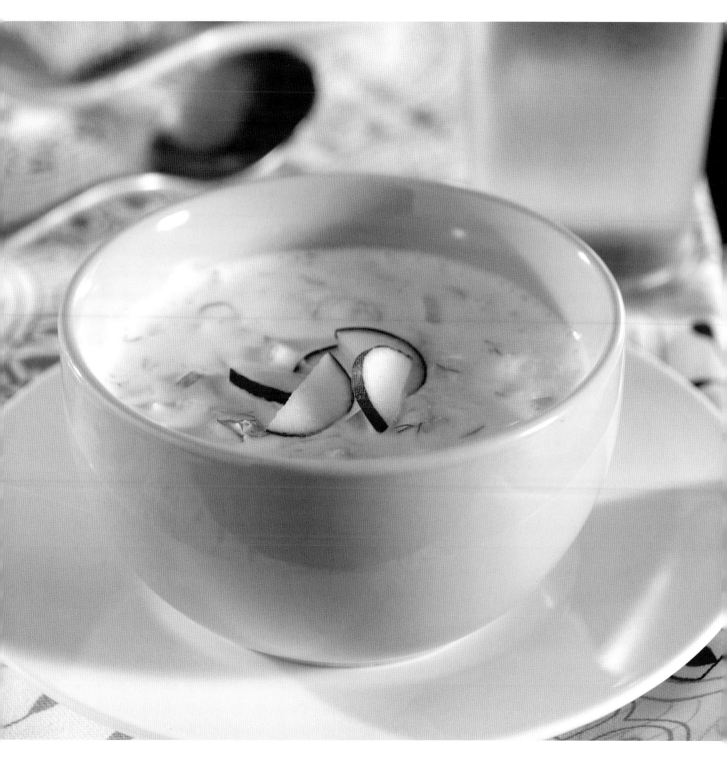

CHEESY BROCCOLI SOUP

½ teaspoon olive oil

¼ cup finely chopped onion

1 cup chicken broth

3 cups small broccoli florets or thawed frozen chopped broccoli

½ cup whipping cream

⅛ teaspoon ground red pepper

2 ounces cubed pasteurized process cheese product

¼ cup sour cream

⅛ teaspoon salt

1 Heat oil in medium saucepan over medium-high heat. Add onion; cook and stir 4 minutes or until translucent.

2 Add broth; bring to a boil over high heat. Add broccoli; return to a boil. Reduce heat to low; cover and simmer 5 minutes or until broccoli is tender.

3 Whisk in cream and red pepper. Remove from heat; stir in cheese until melted. Stir in sour cream and salt.

MAKES 2 SERVINGS

PER SERVING

CALORIES 400, TOTAL FAT 34g, CARBS 12g, NET CARBS 9g, DIETARY FIBER 3g, PROTEIN 11g

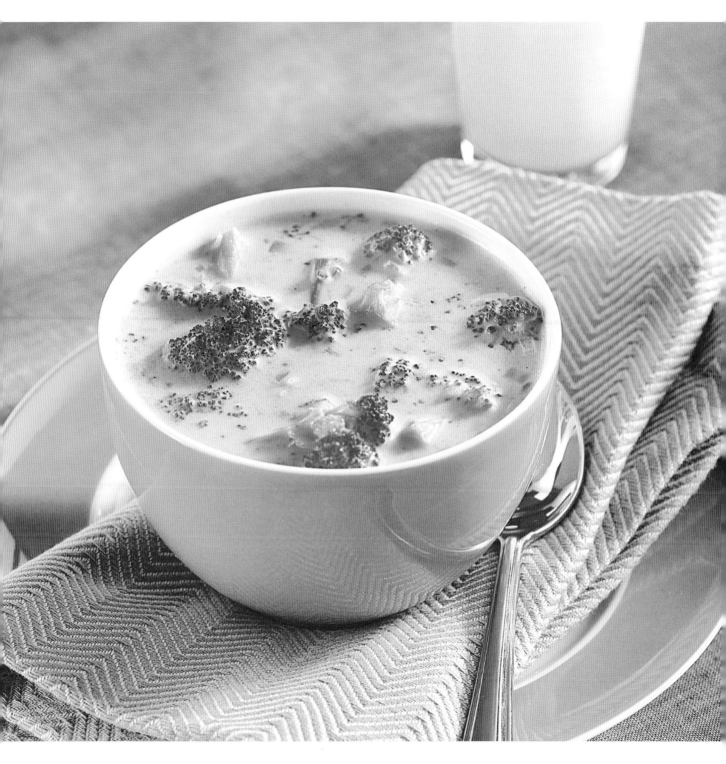

CREAM OF AVOCADO SOUP

6 medium avocados,
   cut into halves and
   pits removed

   Lemon juice

2 cups vegetable
   broth, divided

4 eggs*

4 cups whole milk,
   divided

½ teaspoon salt

¼ teaspoon white
   pepper

3 cups sour cream,
   divided

   Black caviar and
   ground red pepper
   (optional)

*Use clean, uncracked
eggs.

1 Scoop out flesh of avocados leaving ¼-inch shell; set aside avocado flesh. Lightly sprinkle insides of shells with lemon juice to prevent browning. Cover; refrigerate.

2 Process avocado flesh and 1 cup broth in small batches in food processor or blender until smooth. Transfer to large bowl; set aside.

3 In top of double boiler, beat eggs with 2 cups milk. Heat slowly over hot, not boiling, water; stir until mixture is thick enough to coat back of spoon. Remove from heat; stir in remaining 1 cup broth. Let stand at room temperature until cool.

4 Stir cooled egg mixture, salt and white pepper into avocado mixture. Mix in 2 cups sour cream, stirring until smooth. Add remaining 2 cups milk. Process soup in small batches in food processor or blender until smooth. Adjust seasonings. Cover; refrigerate until very cold.

5 To serve, pour cold soup into avocado shells. Top each portion with about 1 tablespoon of the remaining 1 cup sour cream. Garnish, if desired.

MAKES 12 SERVINGS

PER SERVING

CALORIES 360, TOTAL FAT 31g, CARBS 15g, NET CARBS 8g, DIETARY FIBER 7g, PROTEIN 9g

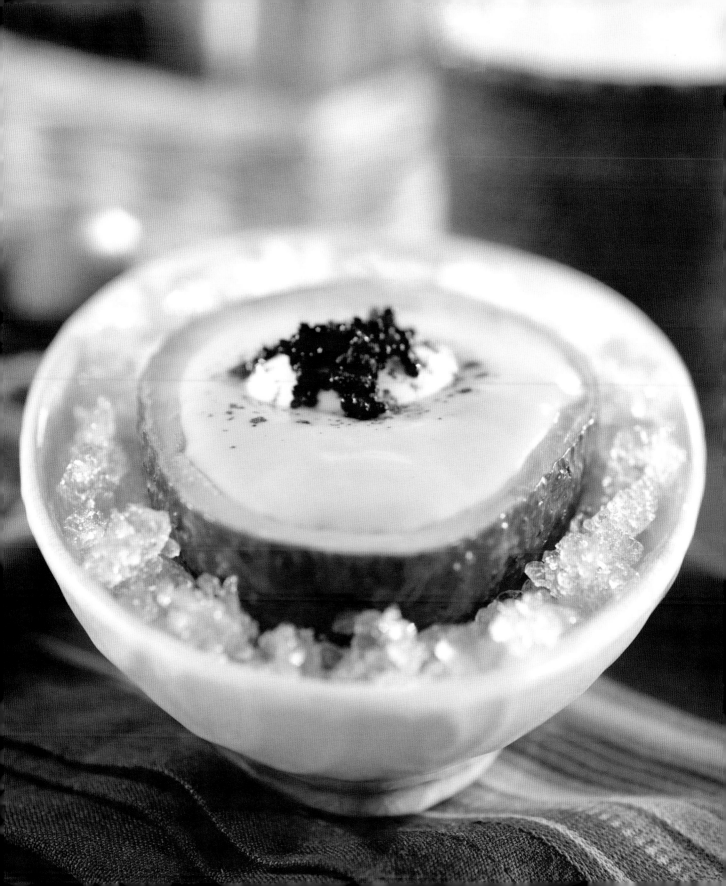

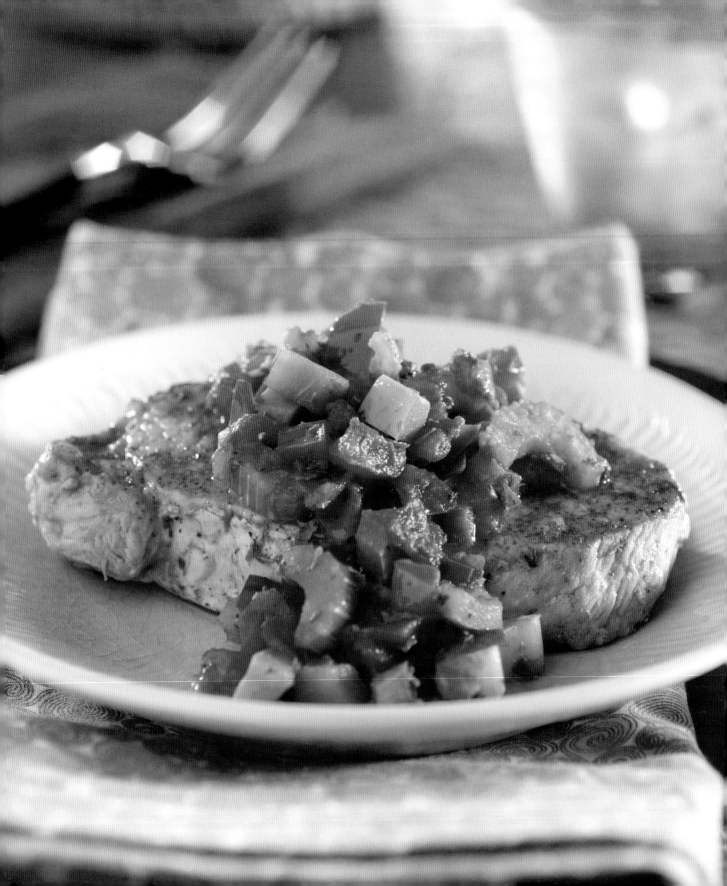

MEAT

ZESTY SKILLET PORK CHOPS

- 1 teaspoon chili powder
- ½ teaspoon salt, divided
- 4 lean boneless pork chops (about 1¼ pounds), well trimmed
- 2 cups diced tomatoes
- 1 cup chopped green, red or yellow bell pepper
- ¾ cup thinly sliced celery
- ½ cup chopped onion
- 1 teaspoon dried thyme
- 1 tablespoon hot pepper sauce
- 2 tablespoons finely chopped fresh parsley

1 Rub chili powder and ¼ teaspoon salt evenly over one side of pork chops.

2 Combine tomatoes, bell pepper, celery, onion, thyme and hot pepper sauce in medium bowl; mix well.

3 Spray large nonstick skillet with nonstick cooking spray; heat over medium-high heat. Add pork, seasoned side down; cook 1 minute. Turn pork. Top with tomato mixture; bring to a boil. Reduce heat to low. Cover; cook 25 minutes or until pork is tender and tomato mixture has thickened.

4 Transfer pork to serving plates. Bring tomato mixture to a boil over high heat; cook 2 minutes or until most liquid has evaporated. Remove from heat; stir in parsley and remaining ¼ teaspoon salt. Spoon sauce over pork.

MAKES 4 SERVINGS

PER SERVING

CALORIES 172, **TOTAL FAT** 7g, **CARBS** 9g, **NET CARBS** 6g, **DIETARY FIBER** 3g, **PROTEIN** 20g

ASPARAGUS STUFFED FLANK STEAK

¼ cup prepared garlic and herb cheese spread

2 pounds flank steak, butterflied, opened

2 tablespoons minced onion

15 thin fresh asparagus spears

Salt and black pepper

1 Preheat oven to 350°F. Spread cheese over steak; sprinkle with onion. Place asparagus side by side in single row over cheese. Roll tightly and secure steak with string or toothpicks. Season outside of roll with salt and pepper; place in roasting pan.

2 Roast 1 hour 15 minutes to 1 hour 30 minutes or until desired doneness. Remove from oven and let stand 10 minutes before slicing.

MAKES 6 SERVINGS

PER SERVING

CALORIES 250, **TOTAL FAT** 11g, **CARBS** 3g, **NET CARBS** 2g, **DIETARY FIBER** 1g, **PROTEIN** 34g

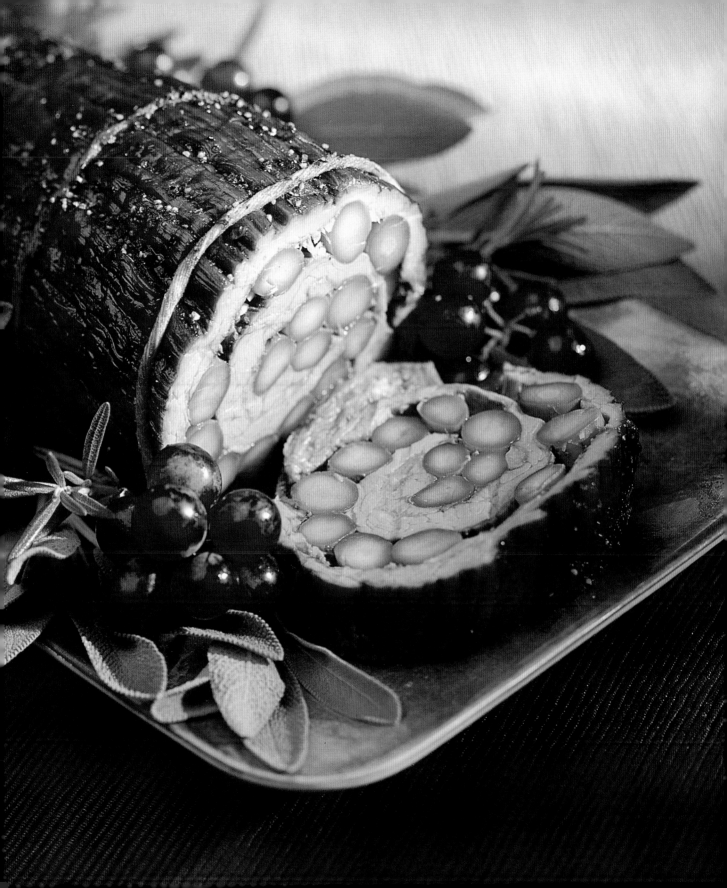

STEAK FAJITAS

¼ cup lime juice

¼ cup soy sauce

4 tablespoons vegetable oil, divided

2 tablespoons Worcestershire sauce

2 cloves garlic, minced

½ teaspoon ground red pepper

1 pound flank steak, skirt steak or top sirloin

1 medium yellow onion, halved and cut into ¼-inch slices

1 green bell pepper, cut into ¼-inch strips

1 red bell pepper, cut into ¼-inch strips

Lime wedges (optional)

Pico de gallo, guacamole, sour cream, shredded lettuce and shredded Cheddar cheese (optional)

1 Combine lime juice, soy sauce, 2 tablespoons oil, Worcestershire sauce, garlic and ground red pepper in medium bowl; mix well. Remove ¼ cup marinade to large bowl. Place steak in large resealable food storage bag. Pour remaining marinade over steak; seal bag and turn to coat. Marinate in refrigerator at least 2 hours or overnight. Add onion and bell peppers to bowl with ¼ cup marinade; toss to coat. Cover and refrigerate until ready to use.

2 Remove steak from marinade; discard marinade and wipe off excess from steak. Heat 1 tablespoon oil in large skillet (preferably cast iron) over medium-high heat. Cook steak about 4 minutes per side for medium rare or to desired doneness. Remove to cutting board; tent with foil and let rest 10 minutes.

3 Meanwhile, heat remaining 1 tablespoon oil in same skillet over medium-high heat. Add vegetable mixture; cook about 8 minutes or until vegetables are crisp-tender and beginning to brown in spots, stirring occasionally. (Cook in 2 batches if necessary; do not pile vegetables in skillet.)

4 Cut steak into thin slices across the grain. Serve with vegetables, lime wedges and desired toppings.

MAKES 4 SERVINGS

PER SERVING

CALORIES 310, **TOTAL FAT** 20g, **CARBS** 7g, **NET CARBS** 6g, **DIETARY FIBER** 1g, **PROTEIN** 26g

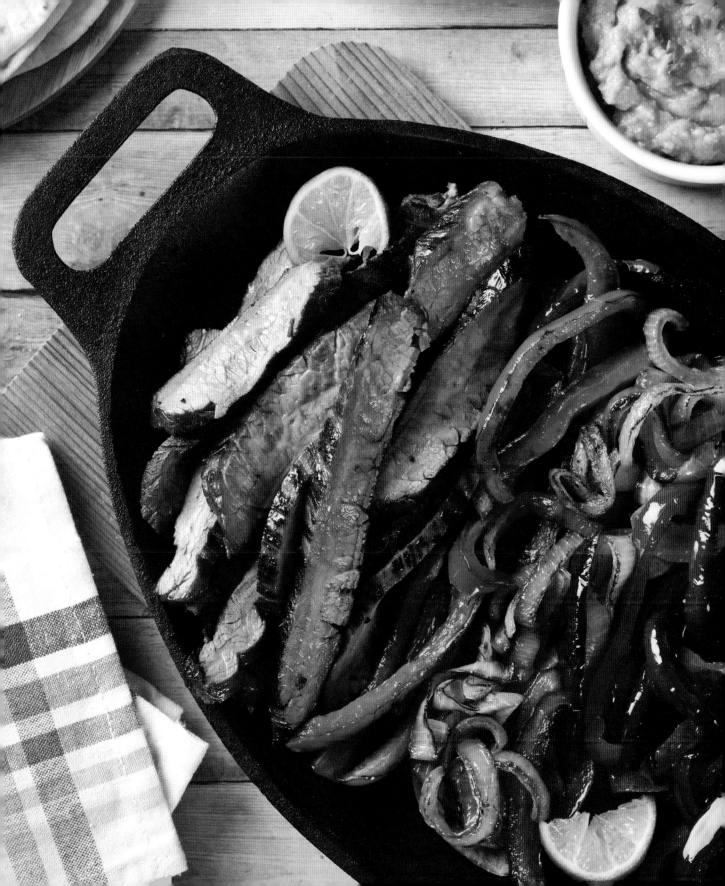

PHILLY CHEESE STEAKS

2 tablespoons canola oil, divided

1 green bell pepper

1 medium onion, peeled and thinly sliced

½ teaspoon salt, divided

½ teaspoon black pepper, divided

¼ teaspoon red pepper flakes (optional)

1 pound boneless beef rib-eye steaks, sliced ¼ inch thick

4 slices American cheese

1 Heat 1 tablespoon oil in large nonstick skillet. Add bell pepper and onion; cook and stir over high heat 3 minutes or until tender. Sprinkle with ¼ teaspoon salt, ¼ teaspoon black pepper and red pepper flakes, if desired. Divide among 4 plates.

2 Heat remaining 1 tablespoon oil in same skillet. Sprinkle steaks with remaining ¼ teaspoon salt and ¼ teaspoon black pepper. Add steak to skillet; sprinkle with additional salt and pepper. Cook and stir 3 minutes or until desired degree of doneness. Top with cheese; cook 1 minute or until cheese is melted. Place steak on vegetables.

MAKES 4 SERVINGS

PER SERVING

CALORIES 294, **TOTAL FAT** 16g, **CARBS** 6g, **NET CARBS** 5g, **DIETARY FIBER** 1g, **PROTEIN** 30g

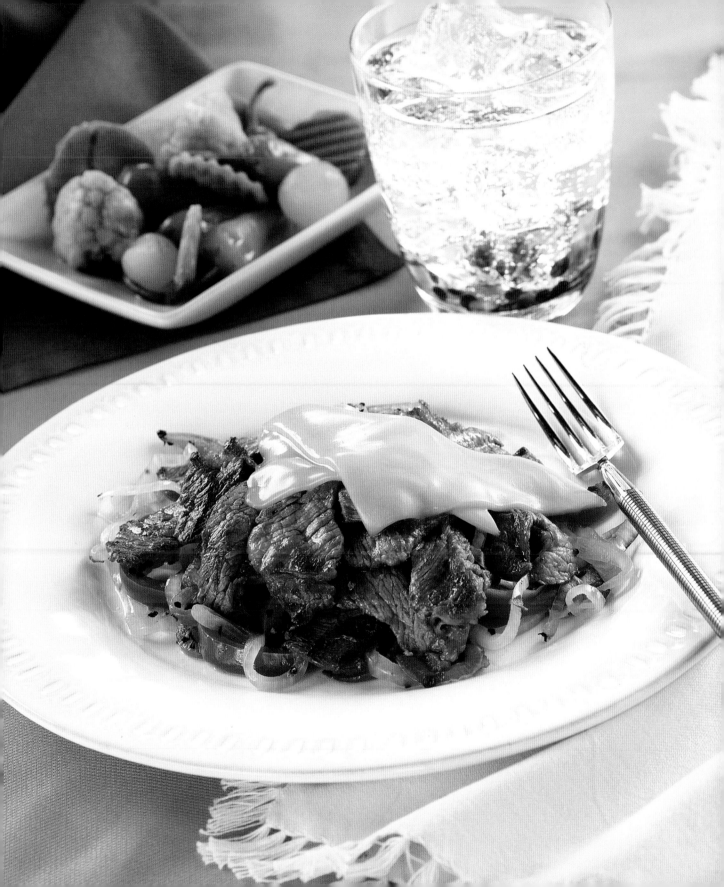

LONDON BROIL WITH MARINATED VEGETABLES

¾ cup olive oil

¾ cup red wine

2 tablespoons finely chopped shallots

2 tablespoons red wine vinegar

2 teaspoons minced garlic

½ teaspoon salt

½ teaspoon dried thyme

½ teaspoon dried oregano

½ teaspoon dried basil

½ teaspoon black pepper

2 pounds top round London broil (1½ inches thick)

1 medium red onion, cut into ¼-inch-thick slices

1 package (8 ounces) sliced mushrooms

1 medium red bell pepper, cut into strips

1 medium zucchini, cut into ¼-inch-thick slices

1 Whisk oil, wine, shallots, vinegar, garlic, salt, thyme, oregano, basil and black pepper in medium bowl until well blended. Combine London broil and ¾ cup marinade in large resealable food storage bag. Seal bag; turn to coat. Marinate in refrigerator at least 1 hour or up to 24 hours, turning bag once or twice.

2 Combine onion, mushrooms, bell pepper, zucchini and remaining marinade in separate large food storage bag. Seal bag; turn to coat. Refrigerate at least 1 hour or up to 24 hours, turning bag once or twice.

3 Preheat broiler. Remove beef from marinade and place on broiler pan; discard marinade. Broil 4 to 5 inches from heat about 9 minutes per side or until desired doneness. Let stand 10 minutes. Thinly slice beef.

4 Meanwhile, drain vegetables and arrange on broiler pan; discard marinade. Broil 4 to 5 inches from heat about 9 minutes or until edges of vegetables just begin to brown. Serve beef with vegetables.

MAKES 6 SERVINGS

PER SERVING

CALORIES 385, **TOTAL FAT** 22g, **CARBS** 6g, **NET CARBS** 4g, **DIETARY FIBER** 2g, **PROTEIN** 37g

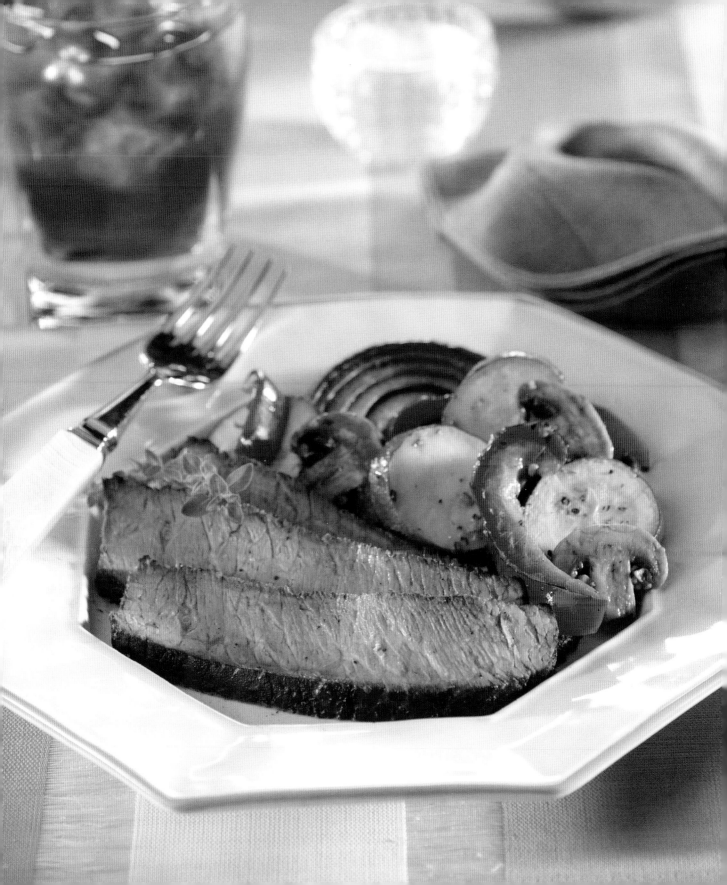

RIB EYE STEAKS WITH CHILI BUTTER

½ cup (1 stick) butter, softened

2 teaspoons chili powder

1 teaspoon minced garlic

1 teaspoon Dijon mustard

⅛ teaspoon ground red pepper or chipotle chile pepper

1 teaspoon black pepper

Salt

4 beef rib eye steaks

1 tablespoon olive oil

1 Beat butter, chili powder, garlic, mustard and red pepper in medium bowl until smooth. Place mixture on sheet of waxed paper. Roll mixture back and forth into 6-inch log using waxed paper. If butter is too soft, refrigerate up to 30 minutes. Wrap with waxed paper; refrigerate at least 1 hour or up to 2 days.

2 Season steaks with black pepper and salt. Heat oil in large cast-iron skillet over medium-high heat. Add steaks; cook 5 minutes per side or to desired doneness.

3 Slice chili butter and serve with steaks.

MAKES 4 SERVINGS

PER SERVING

CALORIES 500, **TOTAL FAT** 37g, **CARBS** 2g, **NET CARBS** 1g, **DIETARY FIBER** 1g, **PROTEIN** 40g

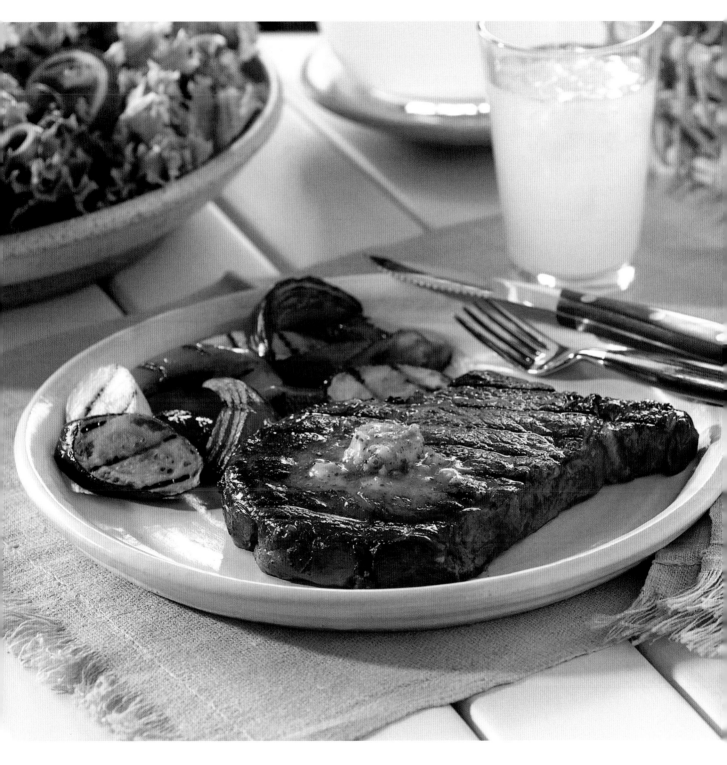

PORK MEDALLIONS WITH MARSALA

1 pound pork tenderloin, cut into ½-inch slices

Salt and black pepper

2 tablespoons olive oil

1 clove garlic, minced

½ cup sweet marsala wine

2 tablespoons chopped fresh parsley

1 Season pork with salt and pepper. Heat oil in large skillet over medium-high heat. Add pork; cook 3 minutes on each side or until browned. Remove from skillet. Reduce heat to medium.

2 Add garlic to skillet; cook and stir 1 minute. Add wine and pork; cook 3 minutes or until pork is barely pink in center. Remove pork from skillet. Stir in parsley. Simmer wine mixture 2 to 3 minutes or until slightly thickened. Serve over pork.

MAKES 4 SERVINGS

PER SERVING

CALORIES 218, **TOTAL FAT** 10g, **CARBS** 1g, **NET CARBS** 0g, **DIETARY FIBER** 1g, **PROTEIN** 24g

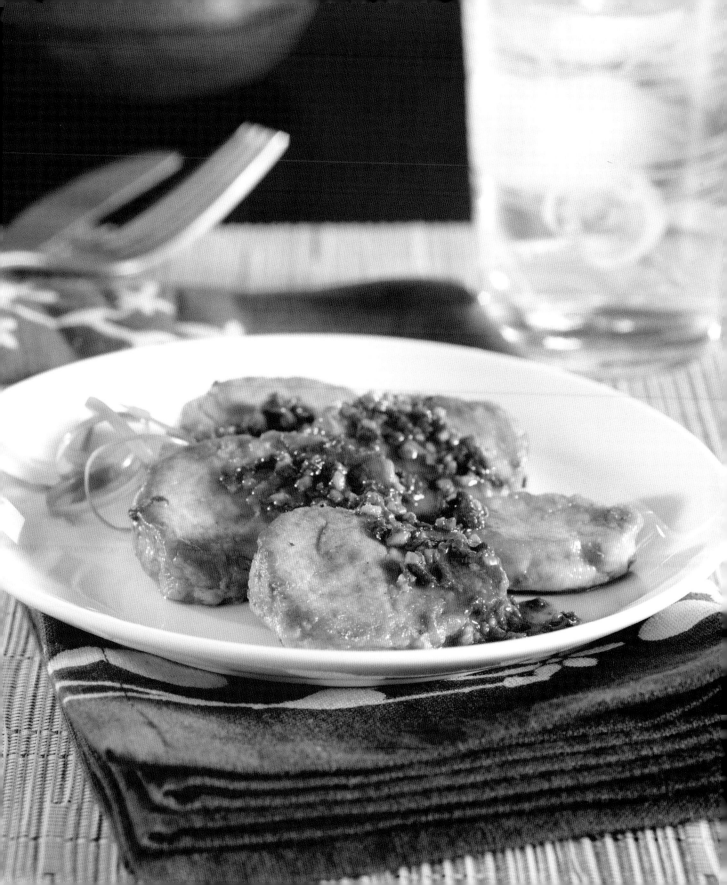

BACON AND ONION BRISKET

6 slices bacon, cut crosswise into ½-inch strips

1 flat-cut boneless beef brisket (about 2½ pounds)

Salt and black pepper

3 medium onions, sliced

2 cans (14 ounces each) beef broth

SLOW COOKER DIRECTIONS

1 Cook bacon in large skillet over medium-high heat 3 minutes. Transfer to slow cooker with slotted spoon.

2 Season brisket with salt and pepper. Sear brisket in hot bacon fat on all sides, turning as it browns. Transfer to slow cooker.

3 Reduce heat to medium. Add sliced onions to skillet. Cook and stir 3 to 5 minutes or until softened. Add to slow cooker. Pour in broth. Cover; cook on HIGH 6 to 8 hours or until meat is tender.

4 Transfer brisket to cutting board and let rest 10 minutes. Thinly slice brisket against the grain; season with salt and pepper, if desired. Spoon bacon, onions and cooking liquid over brisket to serve.

MAKES 6 SERVINGS

PER SERVING

CALORIES 360, **TOTAL FAT** 18g, **CARBS** 5g, **NET CARBS** 4g, **DIETARY FIBER** 1g, **PROTEIN** 45g

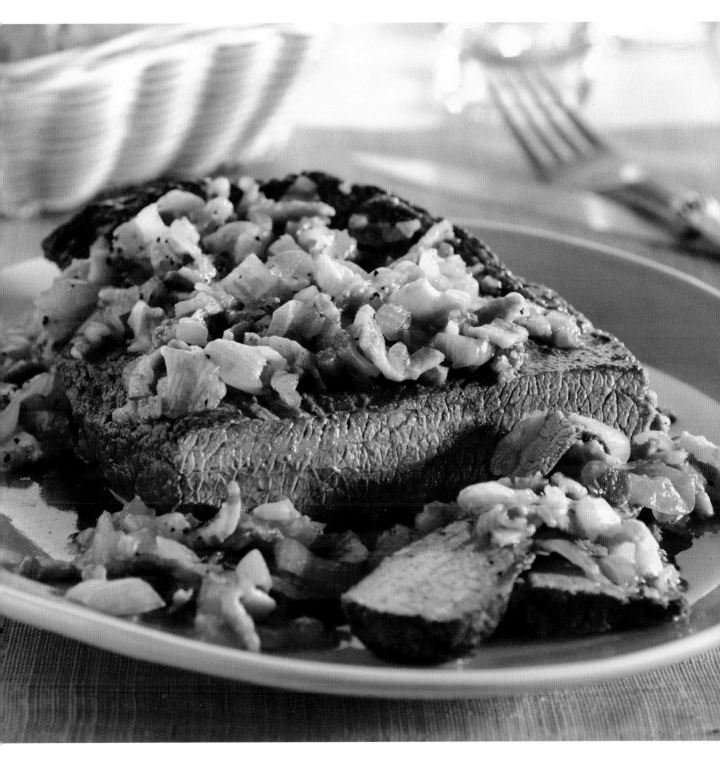

STEAK DIANE WITH CREMINI MUSHROOMS

- 2 beef tenderloin steaks (4 ounces each), cut ¾ inch thick
- ¼ teaspoon black pepper
- ⅓ cup sliced shallots or chopped onion
- 4 ounces cremini mushrooms, sliced *or* 1 (4-ounce) package sliced mixed wild mushrooms
- 1½ tablespoons Worcestershire sauce
- 1 tablespoon Dijon mustard

1 Spray large skillet with nonstick cooking spray; heat over medium-high heat. Add steaks; sprinkle with pepper. Cook 3 minutes per side for medium rare or to desired doneness. Transfer to plate; cover to keep warm.

2 Spray same skillet with cooking spray; place over medium heat. Add shallots; cook and stir 2 minutes. Add mushrooms; cook and stir 3 minutes. Add Worcestershire sauce and mustard; cook 1 minute, stirring frequently.

3 Return steaks and any accumulated juices to skillet; heat through, turning once. Transfer steaks to serving plates; top with mushroom mixture.

MAKES 2 SERVINGS

PER SERVING

CALORIES 270, **TOTAL FAT** 10g, **CARBS** 7g, **NET CARBS** 6g, **DIETARY FIBER** 1g, **PROTEIN** 35g

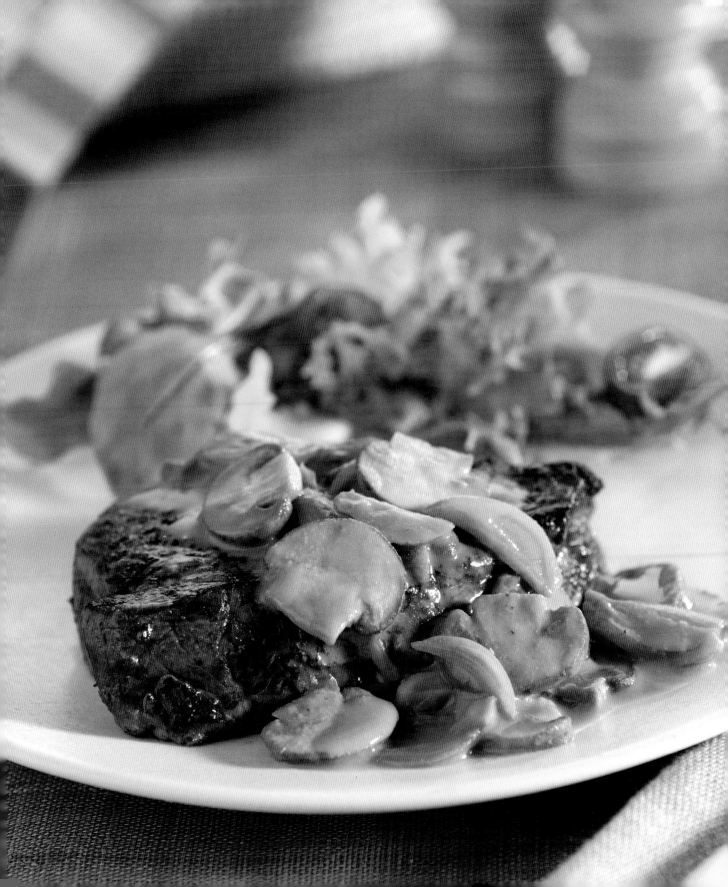

PORK ROAST WITH DIJON TARRAGON GLAZE

⅓ cup chicken or vegetable broth

2 tablespoons Dijon mustard

2 tablespoons lemon juice

1 teaspoon minced fresh tarragon

1½ to 2 pounds boneless pork loin roast, trimmed

1 teaspoon ground paprika

½ teaspoon salt

½ teaspoon black pepper

SLOW COOKER DIRECTIONS

1 For glaze, combine broth, mustard, lemon juice and tarragon in small bowl. Sprinkle roast with paprika, salt and pepper. Place roast in slow cooker. Spoon glaze evenly over roast. Cover; cook on LOW 6 to 8 hours or on HIGH 3 to 4 hours.

2 Remove roast from slow cooker; let stand 15 minutes before slicing.

MAKES 4 SERVINGS

PER SERVING

CALORIES 170, **TOTAL FAT** 6g, **CARBS** 2g, **NET CARBS** 1g, **DIETARY FIBER** 1g, **PROTEIN** 25g

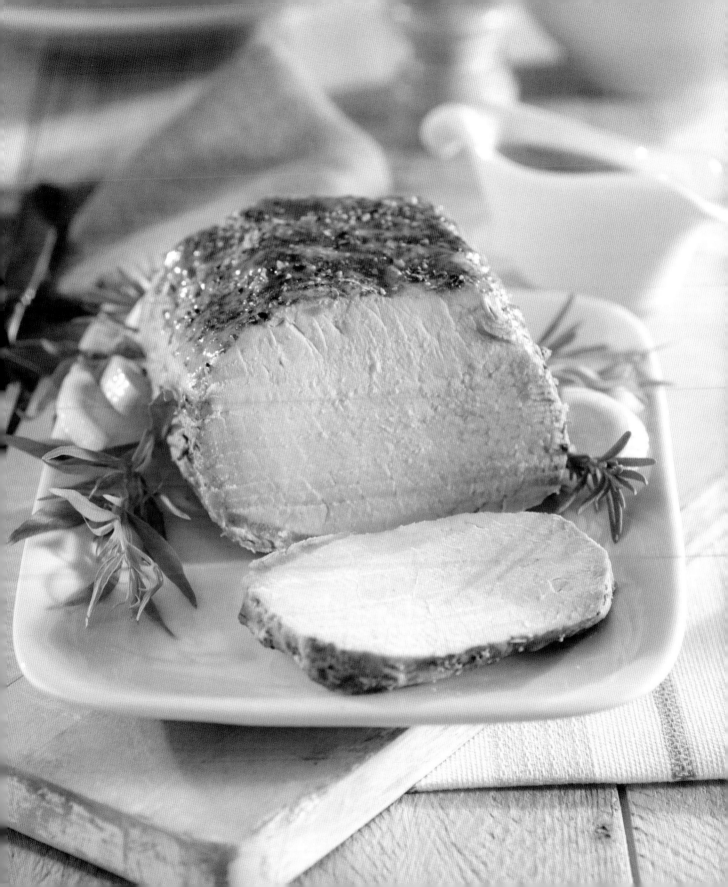

BOLOGNESE-STYLE PORK RAGÙ OVER SPAGHETTI SQUASH

1½ pounds ground pork
1 cup finely chopped celery
½ cup chopped onion
2 cloves garlic, minced
2 tablespoons tomato paste
1 teaspoon Italian seasoning
1 can (about 14 ounces) chicken broth
½ cup half-and-half
1 spaghetti squash (3 to 4 pounds)
½ cup grated Parmesan cheese (optional)

1 Brown pork in large saucepan over medium-high heat, stirring to break up meat. Add celery and onion; cook and stir 5 minutes or until vegetables are tender. Add garlic; cook and stir 1 minute. Stir in tomato paste and Italian seasoning.

2 Stir in broth. Reduce heat. Simmer 10 to 15 minutes, stirring occasionally.

3 Add half-and-half; cook and stir until heated through. Skim off excess fat.

4 Meanwhile, pierce squash several times with knife. Microwave on HIGH 15 minutes or until squash is tender (squash will yield when pressed with finger). Let cool 10 to 15 minutes. Cut in half; scoop out and discard seeds. Separate flesh into strands with fork.

5 Place on serving plates; top with sauce and cheese, if desired.

MAKES 8 SERVINGS

PER SERVING

CALORIES 333, TOTAL FAT 22g, CARBS 15g,
NET CARBS 13g, DIETARY FIBER 2g, PROTEIN 20g

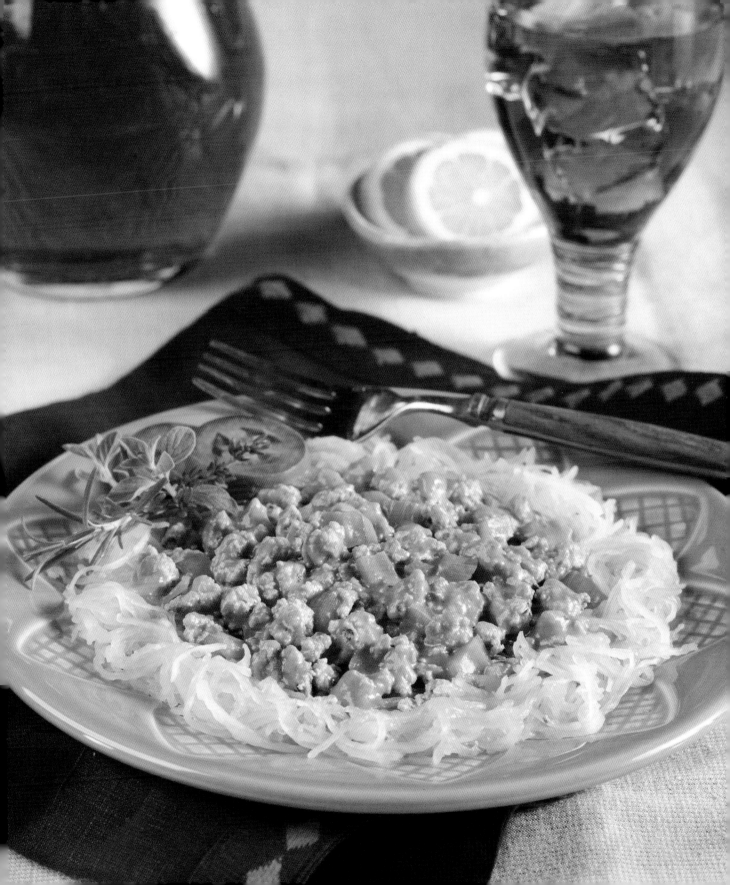

SKIRT STEAK WITH RED PEPPER CHIMICHURRI

- 1 clove garlic, peeled and cut in half
- 1 pound skirt steak, trimmed
- ¼ teaspoon salt
- ½ teaspoon black pepper, divided
- 1 cup diced roasted red pepper
- 1 shallot, minced
- 1 tablespoon capers
- 1½ tablespoons olive oil
- 1 tablespoon white wine vinegar
- 1 clove garlic, minced

1 Preheat broiler. Spray broiler rack with nonstick cooking spray. Rub garlic clove over both sides steak. Season with salt and ¼ teaspoon black pepper. Place steak on broiler rack. Broil steak, 4 inches from heat source, 4 to 5 minutes per side or until desired doneness.

2 For chimichurri sauce, combine red pepper, shallot, capers, oil, vinegar, minced garlic and remaining ¼ teaspoon black pepper in small bowl.

3 Thinly slice steak against the grain; arrange on serving platter. Top with chimichurri sauce or serve separately.

MAKES 4 SERVINGS

PER SERVING

CALORIES 290, **TOTAL FAT** 19g, **CARBS** 5g, **NET CARBS** 4g, **DIETARY FIBER** 1g, **PROTEIN** 24g

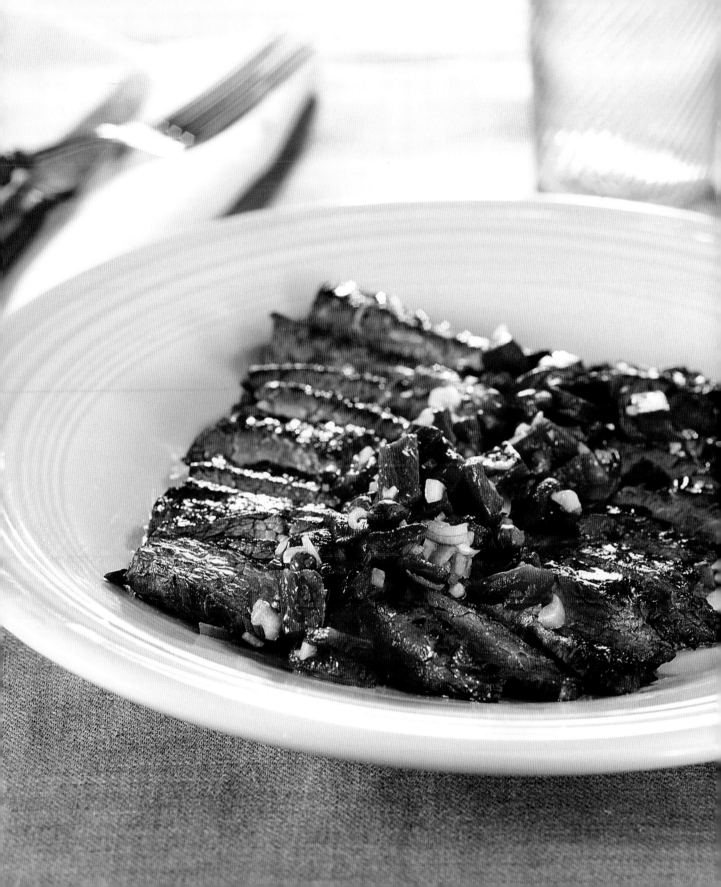

STRIP STEAKS WITH FRESH CHIMICHURRI

½ cup packed fresh basil leaves

⅓ cup plus 1 tablespoon extra virgin olive oil, divided

¼ cup packed fresh parsley

2 tablespoons packed fresh cilantro

2 tablespoons fresh lemon juice

1 clove garlic

1¼ teaspoons salt, divided

½ teaspoon grated orange peel

¼ teaspoon ground coriander

⅛ teaspoon plus ¼ teaspoon black pepper, divided

4 bone-in strip steaks (8 ounces each), about 1 inch thick

¾ teaspoon ground cumin

1 For chimichurri, place basil, ⅓ cup oil, parsley, cilantro, lemon juice, garlic, ½ teaspoon salt, orange peel, coriander and ⅛ teaspoon pepper in food processor or blender; purée.

2 Sprinkle both sides of steaks with remaining ¾ teaspoon salt, cumin and remaining ¼ teaspoon pepper. Heat 1 tablespoon oil in large skillet over medium-high heat. Add steaks; cook 5 minutes per side or to desired doneness. Serve with chimichurri.

MAKES 4 SERVINGS

PER SERVING

CALORIES 630, **TOTAL FAT** 50g, **CARBS** 1g, **NET CARBS** 1g, **DIETARY FIBER** 0g, **PROTEIN** 43g

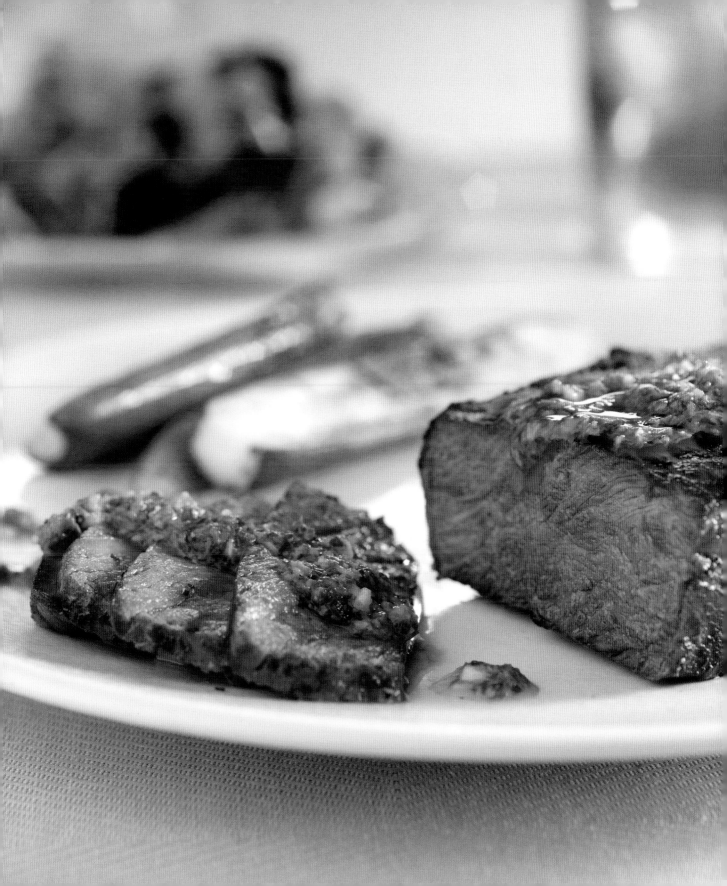

PORK TENDERLOIN WITH SHERRY-MUSHROOM SAUCE

1 to 2 pork tenderloins (1 to 1½ pounds)

Salt and black pepper

1 tablespoon butter

1½ cups chopped button mushrooms or shiitake mushroom caps

2 tablespoons sliced green onion

1 clove garlic, minced

1 tablespoon chopped fresh parsley

½ teaspoon dried thyme

⅓ cup water

1 tablespoon dry sherry

½ teaspoon beef bouillon granules

1 Preheat oven to 375°F. Place pork in large cast iron skillet; season with salt and pepper. Bake 25 to 35 minutes or until thermometer inserted into thickest part of pork registers 145°F. Transfer pork to cutting board. Tent with foil; let stand 5 to 10 minutes.

2 Melt butter in same skillet over medium heat. Add mushrooms, green onion and garlic; cook and stir 3 to 5 minutes or until vegetables are tender. Stir in parsley and thyme; season with additional pepper. Stir in water, sherry and bouillon granules. Cook and stir until sauce boils. Cook and stir 2 minutes more. Slice pork; serve with sauce.

MAKES 4 SERVINGS

PER SERVING

CALORIES 179, **TOTAL FAT** 6g, **CARBS** 4g, **NET CARBS** 3g, **DIETARY FIBER** 1g, **PROTEIN** 26g

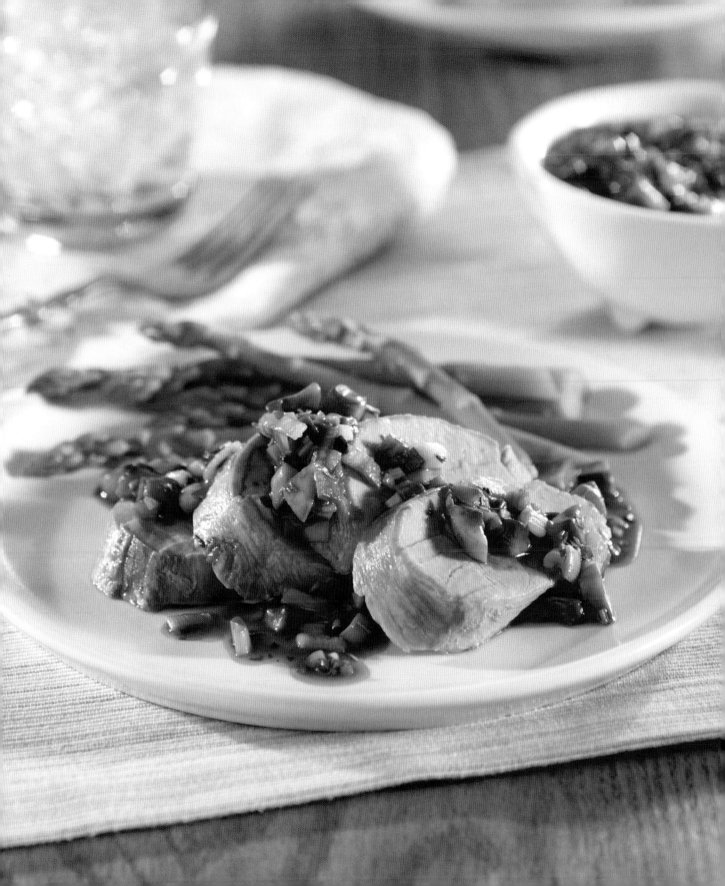

CHINESE PEPPERCORN BEEF

- 2 teaspoons whole black and pink peppercorns*
- 2 teaspoons coriander seeds
- 1 tablespoon peanut or canola oil
- 1 boneless beef top sirloin steak, about 1¼ inches thick (1¼ to 1½ pounds)
- 2 teaspoons dark sesame oil
- ½ cup thinly sliced shallots or sweet onion
- ½ cup chicken broth
- 2 tablespoons soy sauce
- 1 tablespoon dry sherry
- 2 tablespoons thinly sliced green onion or chopped fresh cilantro

Or use all black peppercorns if preferred.

1 Place peppercorns and coriander seeds in small resealable food storage bag; seal bag. Coarsely crush spices using meat mallet or bottom of heavy saucepan. Brush peanut oil over both sides of steak; sprinkle with peppercorn mixture, pressing lightly.

2 Heat large heavy skillet over medium-high heat. Add steak; cook 4 minutes without moving or until seared on bottom. Reduce heat to medium; turn steak and continue cooking 3 to 4 minutes for medium-rare or until desired doneness. Transfer steak to cutting board; tent with foil and let stand while preparing sauce.

3 Add sesame oil to same skillet; heat over medium heat. Add shallots; cook and stir 3 minutes, stirring frequently. Add broth, soy sauce and sherry; simmer 5 to 6 minutes.

4 Carve steak crosswise into thin slices. Spoon sauce over steak; sprinkle with green onion.

MAKES 4 SERVINGS

PER SERVING

CALORIES 330, **TOTAL FAT** 14g, **CARBS** 4g, **NET CARBS** 3g, **DIETARY FIBER** 1g, **PROTEIN** 43g

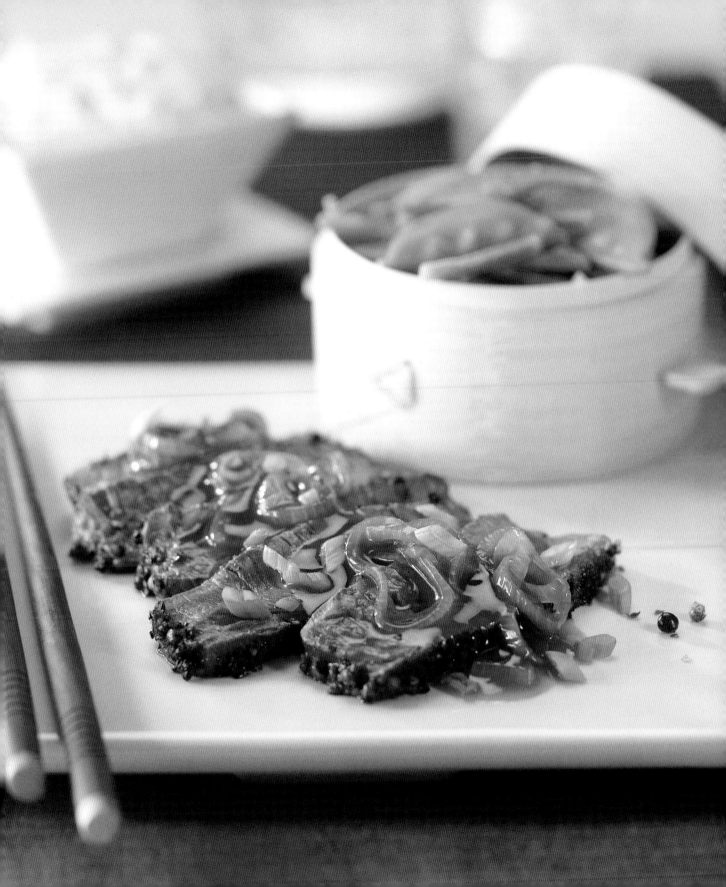

BALSAMIC GRILLED PORK CHOPS

2 tablespoons
  balsamic vinegar

2 tablespoons soy
  sauce

1 teaspoon Dijon
  mustard

⅛ teaspoon red pepper
  flakes

2 boneless pork chops,
  trimmed of fat
  (8 ounces total)

1 Combine vinegar, soy sauce, mustard and red pepper flakes in small bowl. Stir until well blended. Reserve 1 tablespoon marinade; refrigerate until needed.

2 Place pork in large resealable food storage bag. Pour remaining marinade over pork. Seal bag; turn to coat. Refrigerate 2 hours or up to 24 hours.

3 Spray grill pan with nonstick cooking spray; heat over medium-high heat. Remove pork from marinade; discard marinade. Cook pork 4 minutes on each side or until just slightly pink in center. Place on plates; top with reserved 1 tablespoon marinade.

MAKES 2 SERVINGS

PER SERVING

CALORIES 180, **TOTAL FAT** 5g, **CARBS** 4g, **NET CARBS** 3g, **DIETARY FIBER** 1g, **PROTEIN** 26g

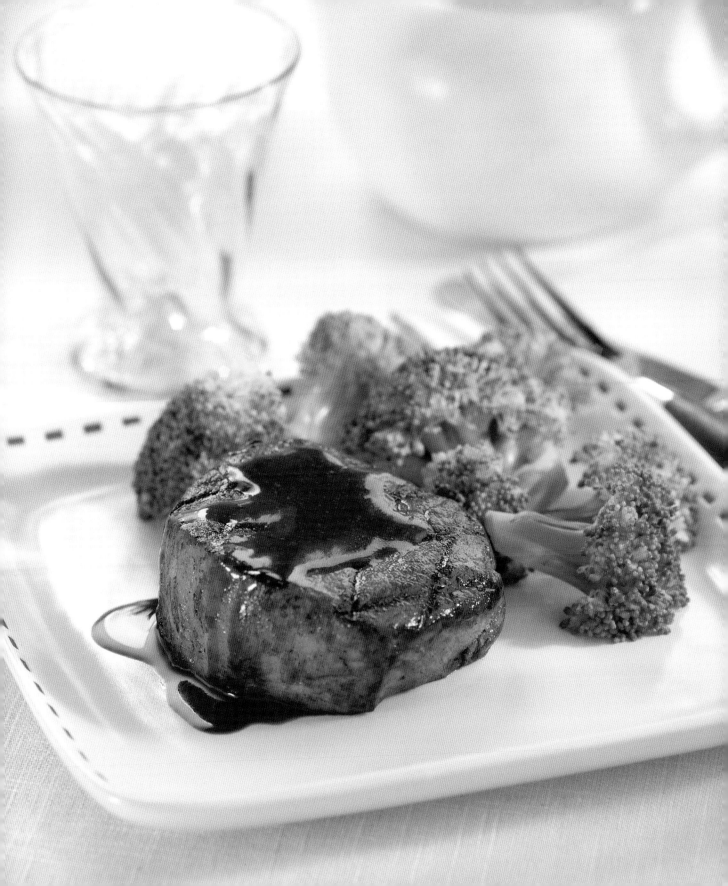

BEEF PATTIES WITH BLUE CHEESE

- 1 pound 95% lean ground beef
- 2 tablespoons steak sauce
- ½ teaspoon salt, divided
- ¼ cup crumbled blue cheese
- 1 teaspoon olive oil
- 8 ounces (about 1½ cups) yellow squash, cut in half lengthwise, then crosswise into ½-inch slices
- 1 medium onion, cut into 8 wedges
- ¼ cup finely chopped fresh parsley

1 Combine beef, steak sauce and ¼ teaspoon salt in small bowl; mix well. Shape into 4 patties.

2 Spray large nonstick skillet with nonstick cooking spray; heat over medium-high heat until hot. Cook patties 4 minutes. Reduce heat to medium. Turn patties; cook 3 to 4 minutes longer or until no longer pink in center (160°F). Transfer to plate. Sprinkle each patty with 1 tablespoon cheese; cover with foil to keep warm.

3 Add oil to same skillet. Add squash and onion; cook and stir 5 to 6 minutes over medium-high heat or until edges of vegetables begin to brown; sprinkle with remaining ¼ teaspoon salt. Spoon vegetables over beef; sprinkle evenly with parsley.

MAKES 4 SERVINGS

PER SERVING

CALORIES 219, **TOTAL FAT** 9g, **CARBS** 6g, **NET CARBS** 5g, **DIETARY FIBER** 1g, **PROTEIN** 27g

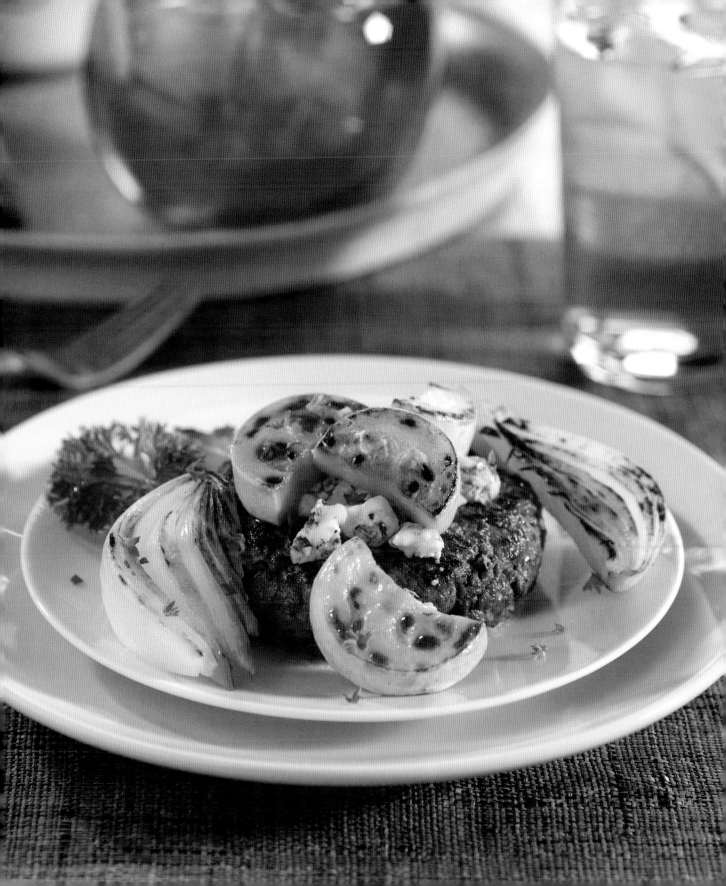

HERBED STANDING RIB ROAST

2 teaspoons kosher salt

1 (4-rib) bone-in standing rib roast (about 9 pounds)

2 tablespoons olive oil

4 cloves garlic, minced

2 teaspoons grated lemon peel

2 tablespoons chopped fresh rosemary

2 tablespoons chopped fresh thyme

2 tablespoons chopped fresh Italian parsley

2 tablespoons chopped fresh oregano

2 teaspoons black pepper

¼ teaspoon red pepper flakes

1 Sprinkle salt over entire roast. Wrap with plastic wrap and refrigerate at least 2 hours or up to 2 days.

2 Combine oil, garlic, lemon peel, rosemary, thyme, parsley, oregano, black pepper and red pepper flakes in small bowl; mix well. Rub paste all over roast. Allow roast to sit at room temperature at least 1 hour or up to 2 hours.

3 Preheat oven to 450°F. Spray roasting pan with nonstick cooking spray (it should be just large enough to fit the roast). Place roast, bone side down, in prepared pan. Roast 25 minutes. *Reduce oven temperature to 350°F.* Roast 1½ to 2 hours or until meat thermometer inserted into thickest part of roast registers 120° to 125°F (rare), or 130° to 140°F (medium-rare). Tent with foil. Let stand 15 to 20 minutes before slicing.

MAKES 16 SERVINGS

PER SERVING

CALORIES 580, **TOTAL FAT** 48g, **CARBS** 1g, **NET CARBS** 1g, **DIETARY FIBER** 0g, **PROTEIN** 35g

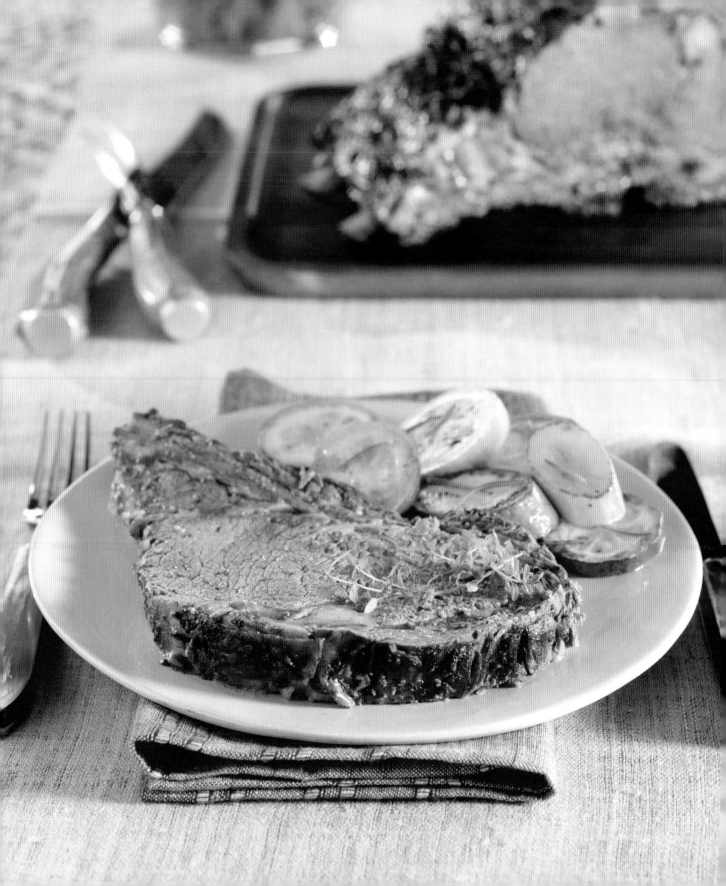

SMOKED SAUSAGE AND CABBAGE

- 1 pound smoked sausage, cut into 2-inch pieces
- 1 tablespoon olive oil
- 6 cups coarsely chopped cabbage
- 1 yellow onion, cut into ½-inch wedges
- 2 cloves garlic, minced
- ¼ teaspoon caraway seeds
- ¼ teaspoon salt
- ¼ teaspoon black pepper

1 Cook and stir sausage in large nonstick skillet over medium-high heat 3 minutes or until browned. Transfer to plate.

2 Heat oil in same skillet. Add cabbage, onion, garlic, caraway seeds, salt and pepper; cook and stir 5 minutes or until onion begins to brown. Add sausage; cover and cook 5 minutes. Remove from heat; let stand 5 minutes.

MAKES 6 SERVINGS

PER SERVING

CALORIES 300, **TOTAL FAT** 24g, **CARBS** 10g, **NET CARBS** 8g, **DIETARY FIBER** 2g, **PROTEIN** 9g

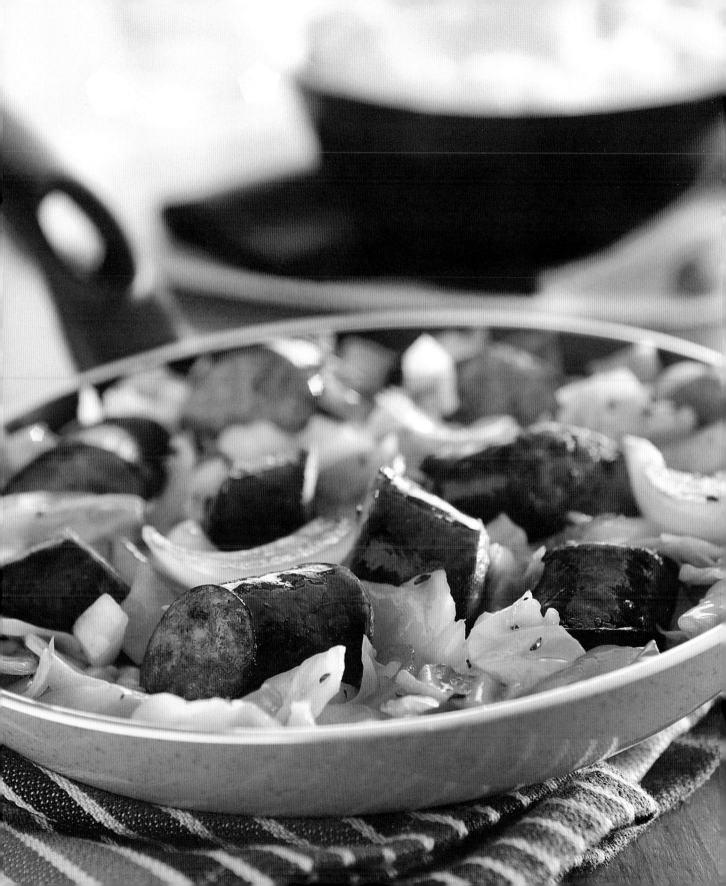

GREEK LAMB WITH TZATZIKI SAUCE

2½ to 3 pounds boneless leg of lamb

8 cloves garlic, divided

¼ cup Dijon mustard

2 tablespoons minced fresh rosemary leaves

2 teaspoons salt

2 teaspoons black pepper

¼ cup plus 2 teaspoons olive oil, divided

1 small seedless cucumber

1 tablespoon chopped fresh mint

1 teaspoon lemon juice

2 cups plain nonfat Greek yogurt or other thick plain yogurt

1 Untie and unroll lamb to lie flat; trim fat.

2 For marinade, mince 4 garlic cloves; place in small bowl. Add mustard, rosemary, salt and pepper; whisk in ¼ cup oil. Spread mixture evenly over lamb, coating both sides. Place lamb in large resealable food storage bag. Seal bag; refrigerate at least 2 hours or overnight, turning several times.

3 Meanwhile for tzatziki sauce, mince remaining 4 garlic cloves and mash to a paste; place in medium bowl. Peel and grate cucumber; squeeze to remove excess moisture. Add cucumber, mint, remaining 2 teaspoons oil and lemon juice to bowl with garlic. Add yogurt; mix well. Season to taste with salt. Refrigerate until ready to serve.

4 Preheat oven to 325°F. Place lamb on rack in roasting pan. Roast about 1½ hours or to desired doneness. Cover loosely with foil; let rest 5 to 10 minutes. (Remove from oven at 140°F for medium. Temperature will rise 5°F while resting.)

5 Slice lamb and serve with tzatziki sauce.

MAKES 4 SERVINGS

PER SERVING

CALORIES 360, **TOTAL FAT** 22g, **CARBS** 6g, **NET CARBS** 6g, **DIETARY FIBER** 0g, **PROTEIN** 32g

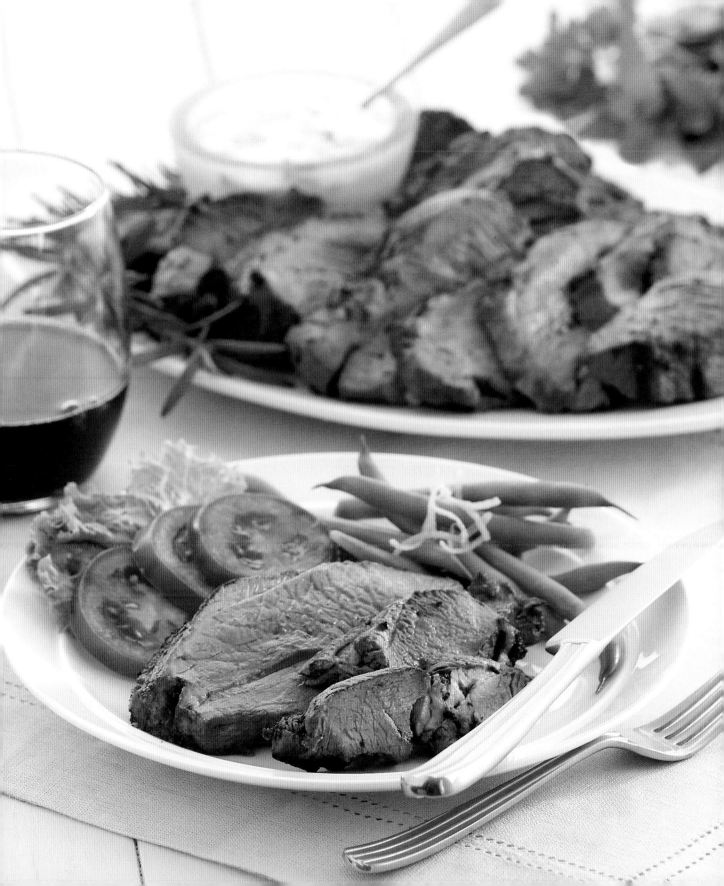

PORK CHOPS BOLOGNESE

4 (¾-inch-thick) bone-in rib pork chops (1 pound)

4 slices prosciutto (4 ounces)

4 slices fontina cheese (4 ounces)

2 teaspoons chopped fresh rosemary leaves

1 teaspoon chopped fresh sage (optional)

2 cloves garlic, minced

Salt and black pepper

2 to 3 tablespoons olive oil

1 Preheat oven to 350°F. Split chops horizontally in half, stopping at bone. Open each chop and arrange 1 slice of prosciutto, folding to fit. Top prosciutto with cheese; trim to fit chops.

2 Sprinkle pork with rosemary, sage, if desired, garlic, salt and pepper. Heat 2 tablespoons oil over medium-high heat in ovenproof skillet large enough to hold chops in single layer. Brown chops 1 to 2 minutes on each side, adding additional oil if needed.

3 Transfer skillet to oven and bake 6 to 10 minutes or until chops are cooked through (160°F).

MAKES 4 SERVINGS

PER SERVING

CALORIES 520, TOTAL FAT 37g, CARBS 1g, NET CARBS 1g, DIETARY FIBER 0g, PROTEIN 44g

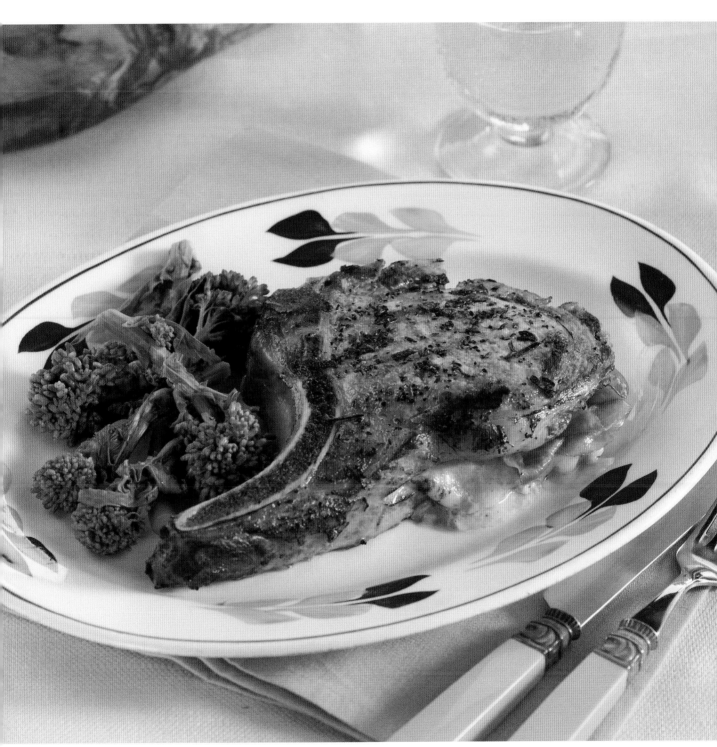

PORK AND PEPPERS MEXICAN-STYLE

2 tablespoons olive oil

½ cup chopped green onions

12 ounces lean pork, cut into ¼-inch pieces

1 *each* red, yellow and green bell peppers, diced (about 2 cups)

1 teaspoon minced garlic

Salt and black pepper

1 cup sliced mushrooms

1 teaspoon ground cumin

1 teaspoon chili powder

½ teaspoon chipotle chili powder (optional)

¼ cup (1 ounce) shredded Cheddar cheese

¼ cup sour cream

1 Heat oil in large skillet over medium high heat. Add green onions; cook and stir 2 minutes. Add pork; cook and stir 5 minutes or until browned. Add bell peppers and garlic; cook and stir 5 minutes or until bell peppers begin to soften.

2 Season mixture in skillet with salt and black pepper. Add mushrooms, cumin, chili powder and chipotle chili powder, if desired. Cook and stir 10 to 15 minutes until pork is cooked through and vegetables are tender. Serve with shredded cheese and sour cream.

MAKES 4 SERVINGS

PER SERVING

CALORIES 271, **TOTAL FAT** 16g, **CARBS** 9g, **NET CARBS** 6g, **DIETARY FIBER** 3g, **PROTEIN** 22g

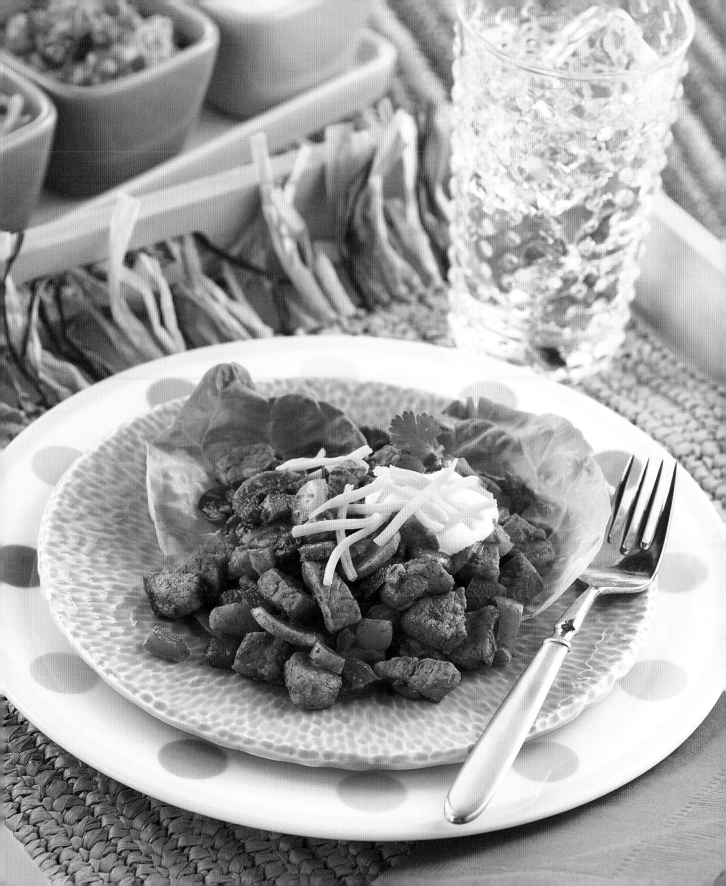

ROSEMARY PORK WITH GARLIC AÏOLI

PORK

- 2 (1-pound) pork tenderloins
- Juice of 2 lemons
- 1 tablespoon olive oil
- ½ teaspoon dried rosemary
- Paprika
- Salt and black pepper

AÏOLI

- ½ cup mayonnaise
- 2 tablespoons olive oil
- 2 tablespoons Dijon mustard
- 1 clove garlic, minced
- ⅛ teaspoon salt

1 Preheat oven to 425°F. Place tenderloins in 13×9-inch baking pan; pour lemon juice over top. Drizzle pork with 1 tablespoon oil; sprinkle with rosemary, paprika, salt and pepper. Let stand 15 minutes to marinate.

2 Meanwhile for aïoli, combine mayonnaise, 2 tablespoons oil, mustard, garlic and ⅛ teaspoon salt in small bowl; cover with plastic wrap and refrigerate until ready to serve. This may be prepared 48 hours in advance.

3 Tuck under thin end of pork. Bake 25 minutes or until barely pink in center (155°F). *Do not overcook.* Remove from oven and let stand 5 minutes. Transfer pork to cutting board and thinly slice.

4 Arrange pork on serving platter. Drizzle with pan juices and serve warm with aïoli.

MAKES 8 SERVINGS

MEAL SUGGESTION

Serve pork and aïoli with mashed cauliflower and roasted brussels sprouts.

PER SERVING

CALORIES 260, **TOTAL FAT** 18g, **CARBS** 1g, **NET CARBS** 1g, **DIETARY FIBER** 0g, **PROTEIN** 24g

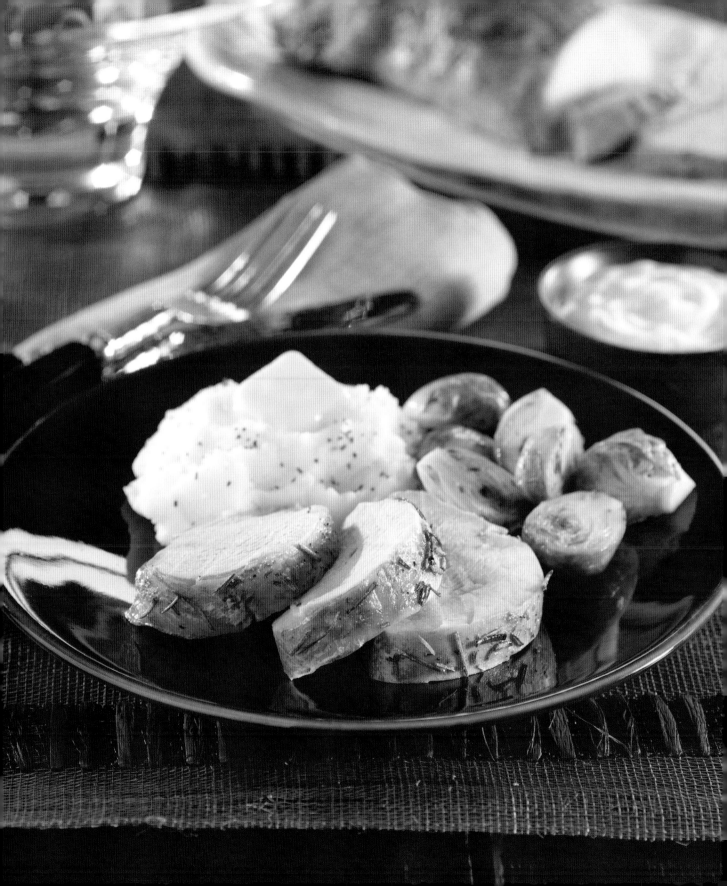

HERB-RUBBED PORK TENDERLOIN WITH MUSTARD SAUCE

1½ teaspoons Italian seasoning

¼ teaspoon black pepper

1 pork tenderloin (about 1½ pounds), trimmed of fat

1½ tablespoons olive oil, divided

1 shallot, minced

1 clove garlic, minced

½ cup chicken broth

⅓ cup whole milk

1 tablespoon Dijon mustard

¼ teaspoon salt

1 Preheat oven to 425°F. Line baking sheet with foil.

2 Combine Italian seasoning and pepper in small bowl; mix well. Rub evenly over pork.

3 Heat 1 tablespoon oil in large cast iron or other ovenproof skillet over medium-high heat. Brown pork on all sides, about 10 minutes. Place on prepared baking sheet.

4 Bake 25 to 30 minutes or until internal temperature reaches 140°F. Transfer to cutting board. Tent with foil and let stand 5 minutes. (Internal temperature will continue to rise 5° to 10°F during stand time.)

5 For sauce, heat remaining ½ tablespoon oil in same skillet over medium heat. Add shallot and garlic; cook and stir 1 minute. Stir in broth, milk, mustard and salt; simmer 2 minutes. Slice pork and serve with sauce.

MAKES 6 SERVINGS

PER SERVING

CALORIES 210, **TOTAL FAT** 10g, **CARBS** 1g, **NET CARBS** 1g, **DIETARY FIBER** 0g, **PROTEIN** 25g

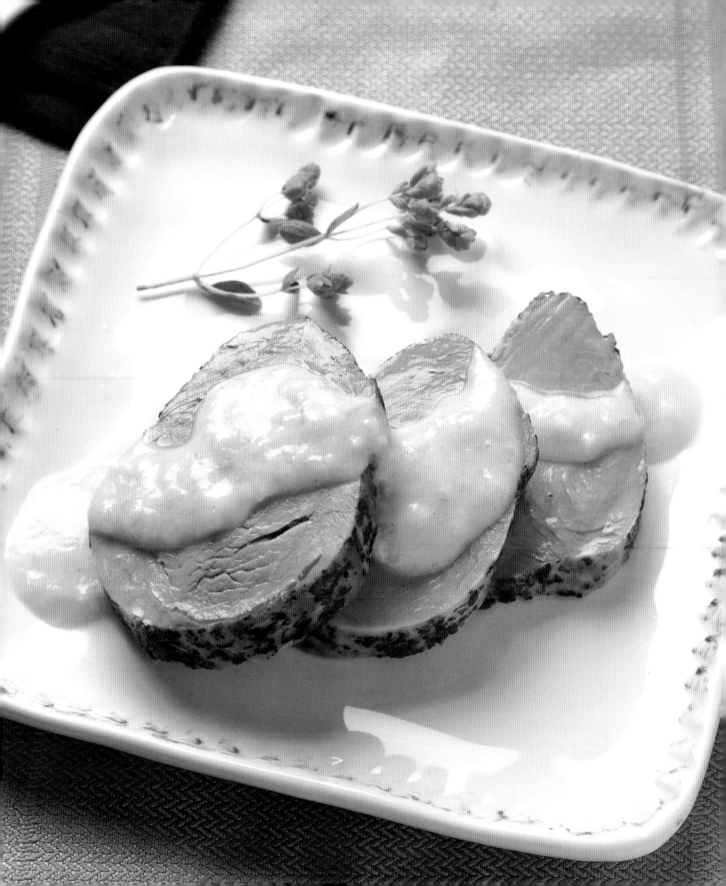

PORK TENDERLOIN OVER RED CABBAGE SLAW

1 pork tenderloin (about 1 pound), trimmed

1 clove garlic, cut into thin slices

1 teaspoon dried oregano

Grated peel of 1 lemon

1 cup plain yogurt

Red Cabbage Slaw (recipe follows)

¼ teaspoon salt

¼ teaspoon black pepper

1 Make small slits in pork in several places with paring knife. Stuff garlic slices, oregano and lemon peel into slits. Place pork in bowl. Add yogurt; spread over all sides of pork to coat. Cover; refrigerate 4 to 6 hours. Prepare slaw.

2 Preheat oven to 425°F. Remove pork from yogurt, scraping off any excess. Sprinkle pork with salt and pepper. Place pork on shallow rack over roasting pan. Roast 45 minutes, turning over once, or until meat thermometer registers 160°F. Remove from heat. Slice ¼ inch thick on diagonal; serve with slaw.

MAKES 4 SERVINGS

PER SERVING

CALORIES 222, **TOTAL FAT** 7g, **CARBS** 11g, **NET CARBS** 10g, **DIETARY FIBER** 1g, **PROTEIN** 28g

RED CABBAGE SLAW

2 cups shredded red cabbage

½ cup chopped green onions, green parts only

2 tablespoons balsamic vinegar

1 tablespoon canola oil

¼ teaspoon salt

¼ teaspoon black pepper

Place cabbage and green onions in medium bowl; toss well. Combine vinegar, oil, salt and pepper in small bowl; stir until well blended. Pour over cabbage; toss to coat. Refrigerate until ready to serve.

MAKES 2 CUPS

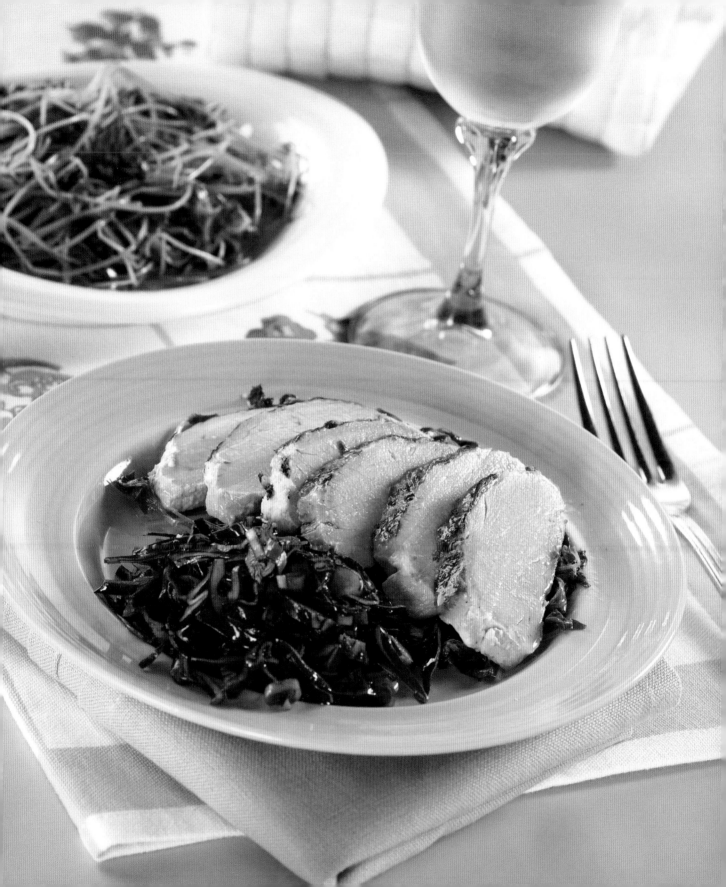

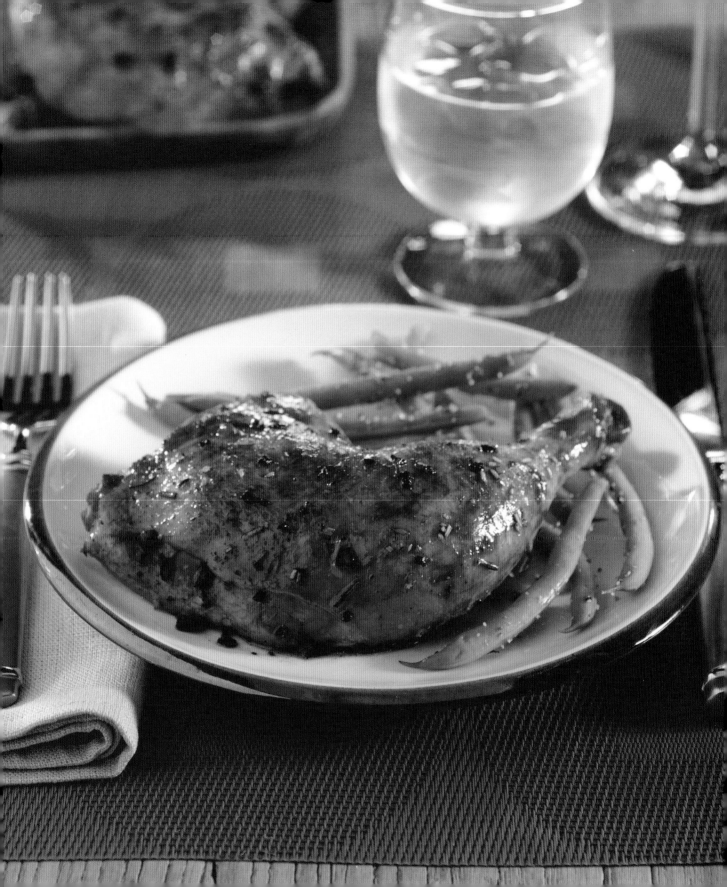

POULTRY

ROASTED ROSEMARY CHICKEN LEGS

¼ cup finely chopped onion

2 tablespoons butter, melted

1 tablespoon chopped fresh rosemary leaves *or* 1 teaspoon dried rosemary

½ teaspoon salt

¼ teaspoon black pepper

2 cloves garlic, minced

4 chicken legs (about 1½ pounds)

¼ cup chicken broth

1 Preheat oven to 375°F.

2 Combine onion, butter, rosemary, salt, pepper and garlic in small bowl; mix well. Gently loosen chicken skin; rub onion mixture under and over skin. Place chicken, skin side up, in small shallow roasting pan. Pour broth over chicken.

3 Roast chicken 50 to 60 minutes or until chicken is browned and cooked through (165°F), basting frequently with pan juices.

MAKES 4 SERVINGS

PER SERVING

CALORIES 263, TOTAL FAT 17g, CARBS 2g, NET CARBS 1g, DIETARY FIBER 1g, PROTEIN 22g

POLLO DIAVOLO (DEVILED CHICKEN)

8 skinless bone-in chicken thighs (2½ to 3 pounds)

¼ cup olive oil

3 tablespoons lemon juice

6 cloves garlic, minced

1 to 2 teaspoons red pepper flakes

3 tablespoons butter, softened

1 teaspoon dried or rubbed sage

1 teaspoon dried thyme

¾ teaspoon coarse salt

¼ teaspoon ground red pepper or black pepper

Lemon wedges

1 Place chicken in large resealable food storage bag. Combine oil, lemon juice, garlic and red pepper flakes in small bowl. Pour mixture over chicken. Seal bag; turn to coat. Refrigerate at least 1 hour or up to 8 hours, turning once.

2 Preheat oven to 375°F. Spray sheet pan with nonstick cooking spray. Place chicken on prepared pan; brush with some of marinade. Bake 40 to 45 minutes or until cooked through (165°F).

3 Meanwhile, combine butter, sage, thyme, salt and ground red pepper in small bowl; mix well. Transfer chicken to serving platter; spread herb butter over chicken. Serve with lemon wedges.

MAKES 4 SERVINGS

PER SERVING

CALORIES 550, TOTAL FAT 34g, CARBS 3g, NET CARBS 3g, DIETARY FIBER 0g, PROTEIN 56g

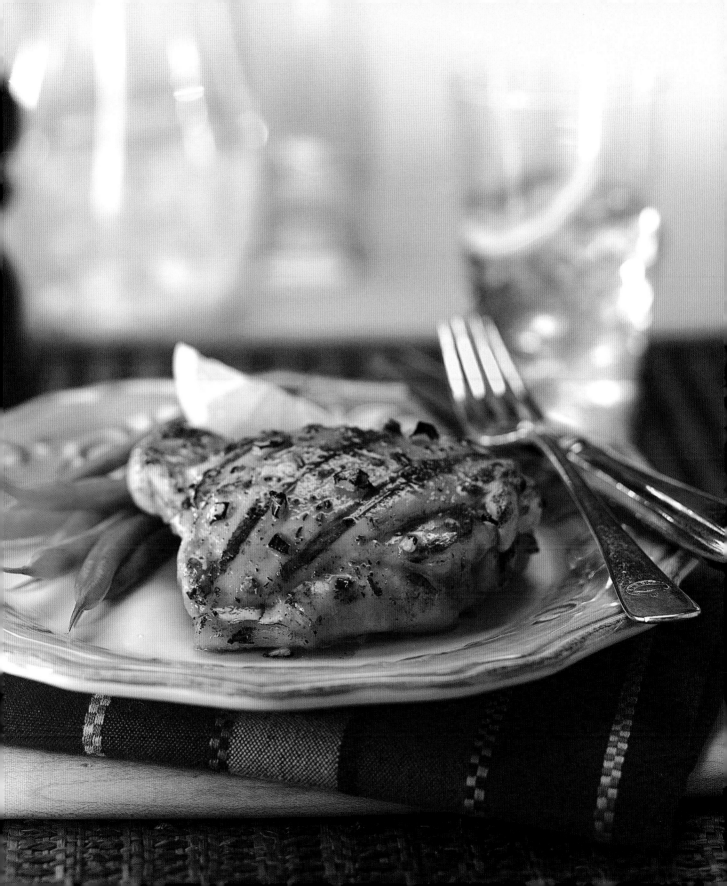

SPICY LEMONY ALMOND CHICKEN

- ½ teaspoon paprika
- ½ teaspoon black pepper
- ¼ teaspoon salt
- 4 boneless skinless chicken breasts (about 1 pound total), flattened to ¼-inch thickness
- 1 ounce slivered almonds, toasted
- ¼ cup water
- 2 tablespoons lemon juice
- 2 tablespoons butter
- 2 teaspoons Worcestershire sauce
- ½ teaspoon grated lemon peel

1 Combine paprika, pepper and salt in small bowl; sprinkle evenly over both sides of chicken.

2 Spray large nonstick skillet with nonstick cooking spray; heat over medium-high heat. Add chicken; cook 3 to 4 minutes per side or until no longer pink in center. Set aside on serving platter. Sprinkle with almonds and cover to keep warm.

3 Add water, lemon juice, butter and Worcestershire sauce to skillet. Cook and stir until reduced to ¼ cup, scraping up browned bits from bottom and side of skillet. Remove from heat. Stir in lemon peel; spoon evenly over chicken.

MAKES 4 SERVINGS

TIP

To pound chicken, place between 2 pieces of plastic wrap. Starting in the center, pound chicken with a meat mallet to reach an even thickness.

PER SERVING

CALORIES 193, TOTAL FAT 7g, CARBS 3g, NET CARBS 2g, DIETARY FIBER 1g, PROTEIN 28g

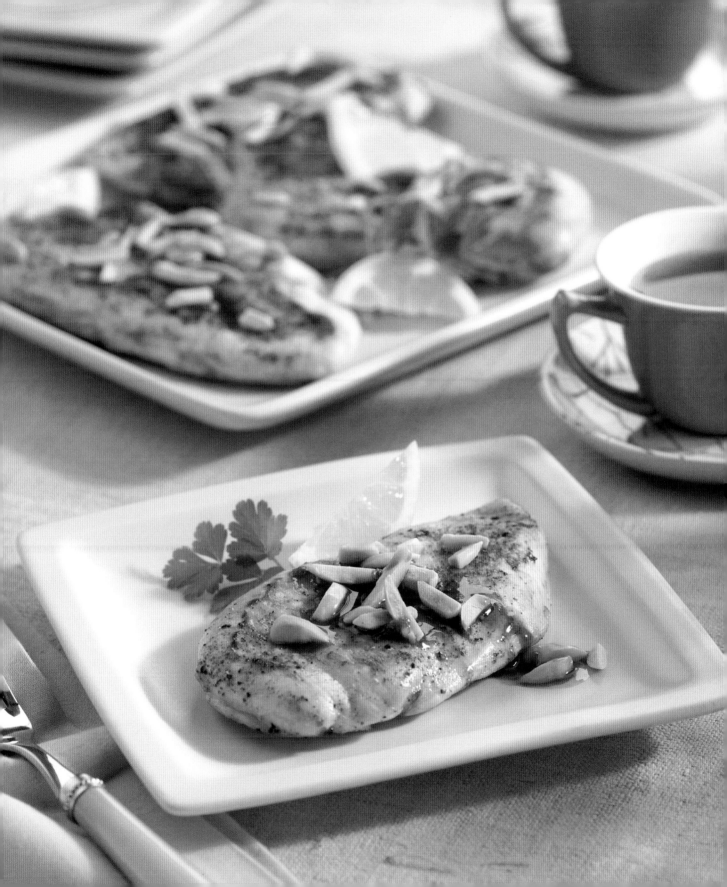

ROAST TURKEY BREAST WITH SPINACH-BLUE CHEESE STUFFING

1 frozen whole boneless turkey breast, thawed (3½ to 4 pounds)

1 package (10 ounces) frozen chopped spinach, thawed and squeezed dry

2 ounces blue cheese or feta cheese

2 ounces reduced-fat cream cheese (Neufchâtel) or regular cream cheese, softened

½ cup finely chopped green onions

1½ tablespoons Dijon mustard

1½ tablespoons dried basil

2 teaspoons dried oregano

Salt, black pepper and paprika

1 Preheat oven to 350°F. Spray roasting pan and rack with nonstick cooking spray.

2 Unroll turkey breast; rinse and pat dry. Place turkey between 2 sheets of plastic wrap or waxed paper. Pound turkey to 1-inch thickness using flat side of meat mallet or rolling pin. Remove and discard skin from one half of turkey breast; turn meat over so skin side (on other half) faces down.

3 Combine spinach, blue cheese, cream cheese, green onions, mustard, basil and oregano in medium bowl; mix well. Spread evenly over turkey breast. Roll up turkey so skin is on top. Tie closed with kitchen string.

4 Carefully place turkey breast on rack; season with salt, pepper and paprika. Roast 1½ hours or until no longer pink in center of breast. Remove from oven; let stand 10 minutes. Remove skin and slice into 14 (¼-inch-thick) slices.

MAKES 14 SERVINGS

PER SERVING

CALORIES 135, TOTAL FAT 4g, CARBS 2g, NET CARBS 1g, DIETARY FIBER 1g, PROTEIN 22g

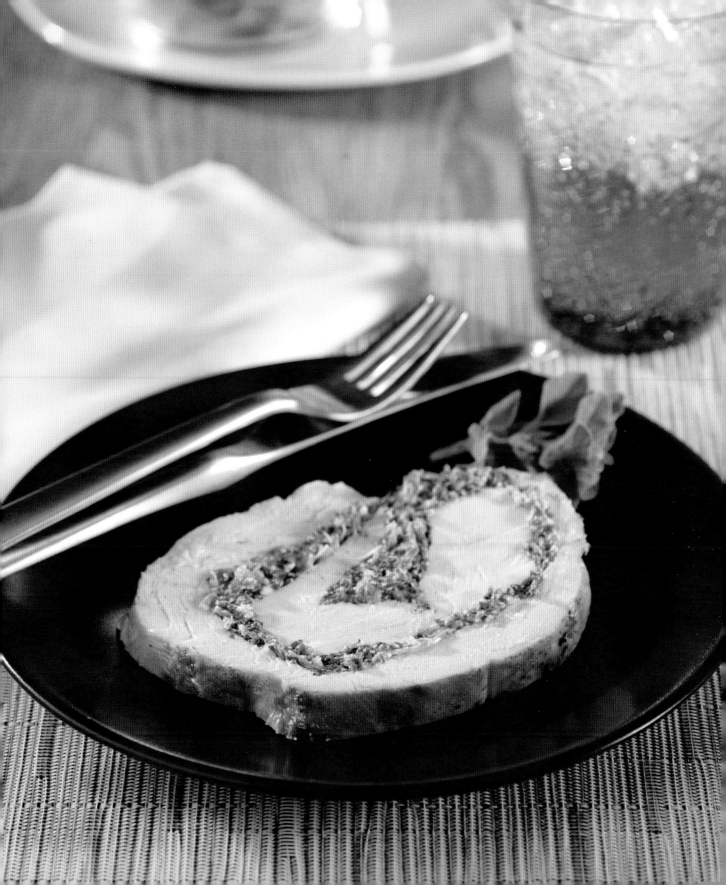

CHICKEN SCARPIELLO

3 tablespoons extra virgin olive oil, divided

1 pound spicy Italian sausage, cut into 1-inch pieces

1 cut-up whole chicken (about 3 pounds)*

1 teaspoon salt, divided

1 large onion, chopped

2 red, yellow or orange bell peppers, cut into ¼-inch strips

3 cloves garlic, minced

½ cup dry white wine

½ cup chicken broth

½ cup coarsely chopped seeded hot cherry peppers

½ cup liquid from cherry pepper jar

1 teaspoon dried oregano

Additional salt and black pepper

¼ cup chopped fresh Italian parsley

*Or purchase 2 bone-in chicken leg quarters and 2 chicken breasts; separate drumsticks and thighs and cut breasts in half.

1 Heat 1 tablespoon oil in large skillet over medium-high heat. Add sausage; cook about 10 minutes or until well browned on all sides, stirring occasionally. Remove sausage from skillet; set aside.

2 Heat 1 tablespoon oil in same skillet. Sprinkle chicken with ½ teaspoon salt; arrange skin side down in single layer in skillet (cook in batches if necessary). Cook about 6 minutes per side or until browned. Remove chicken from skillet; set aside. Drain oil from skillet.

3 Heat remaining 1 tablespoon oil in skillet. Add onion and ½ teaspoon salt; cook and stir 2 minutes or until onion is softened, scraping up any browned bits from bottom of skillet. Add bell peppers and garlic; cook and stir 5 minutes. Stir in wine; cook until liquid is reduced by half. Stir in broth, cherry peppers, cherry pepper liquid and oregano. Season with additional salt and black pepper; bring to a simmer.

4 Return sausage and chicken along with any accumulated juices to skillet. Partially cover skillet and simmer 10 minutes. Uncover and simmer 15 minutes or until chicken is cooked through (165°F). Sprinkle with parsley.

MAKES 4 TO 6 SERVINGS

TIP

If too much liquid remains in the skillet when the chicken is cooked through, remove the chicken and sausage and continue simmering the sauce to reduce it slightly.

PER SERVING

CALORIES 500, TOTAL FAT 35g, CARBS 11g, NET CARBS 10g, DIETARY FIBER 1g, PROTEIN 30g

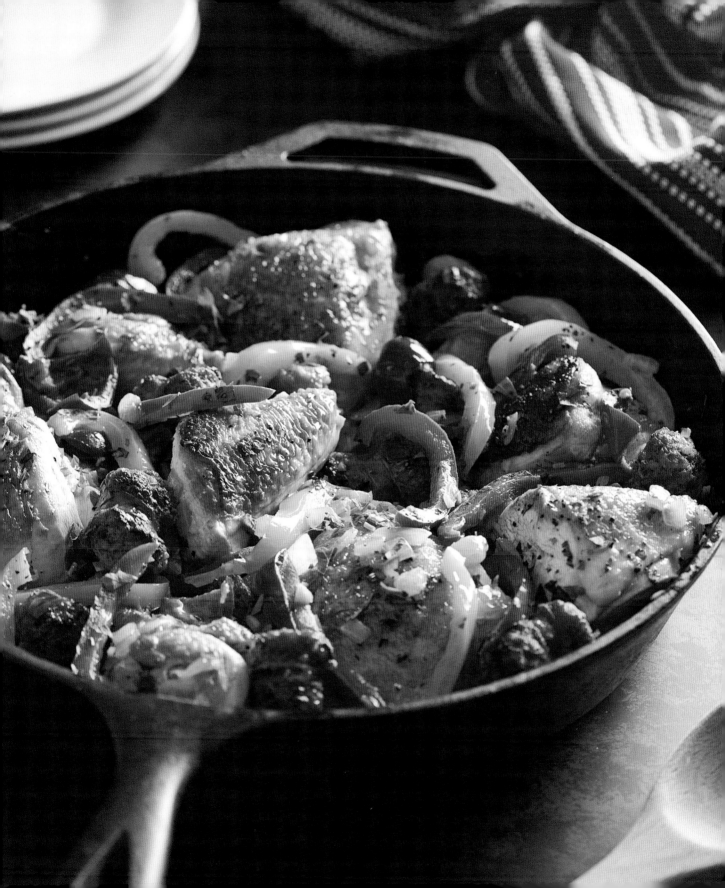

BALSAMIC CHICKEN

1½ teaspoons fresh rosemary leaves, minced, *or* ½ teaspoon dried rosemary

2 cloves garlic, minced

¾ teaspoon black pepper

½ teaspoon salt

6 boneless skinless chicken breasts (about 4 ounces each)

1 tablespoon olive oil

¼ cup balsamic vinegar

1 Combine rosemary, garlic, pepper and salt in small bowl; mix well. Place chicken in large bowl; drizzle chicken with oil and rub with spice mixture. Cover and refrigerate several hours.

2 Preheat oven to 450°F. Spray heavy roasting pan with nonstick cooking spray. Place chicken in pan; bake 10 minutes. Turn chicken over, stirring in 3 to 4 tablespoons water if drippings begin to stick to pan.

3 Bake about 10 minutes or until chicken is golden brown and no longer pink in center. If pan is dry, stir in another 1 to 2 tablespoons water to loosen drippings.

4 Drizzle vinegar over chicken in pan. Place chicken on plates. Stir liquid in pan; drizzle over chicken.

MAKES 6 SERVINGS

PER SERVING

CALORIES 174, TOTAL FAT 5g, CARBS 3g, NET CARBS 2g, DIETARY FIBER 1g, PROTEIN 27g

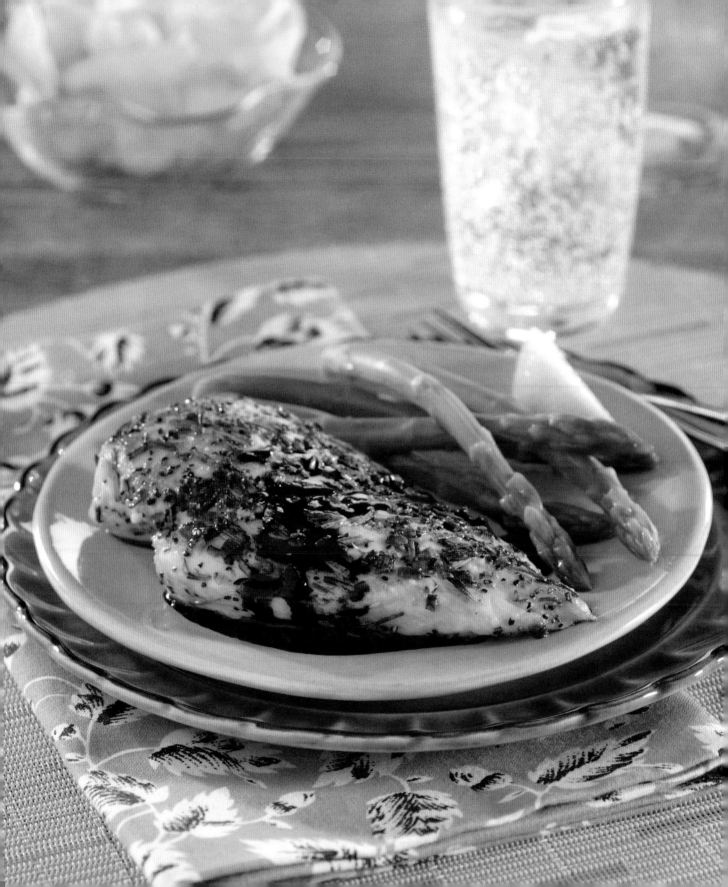

DUCK BREASTS WITH BALSAMIC SAUCE

3 tablespoons balsamic vinegar

2 tablespoons lemon juice

4 boneless duck breasts (6 to 8 ounces each)

Salt and black pepper

1 shallot, minced

1 Combine vinegar and lemon juice in small bowl; mix well.

2 Score skin on duck breasts with tip of sharp knife in crosshatch pattern, being careful to cut only into the fat and not the meat. Season both sides of duck with salt and pepper.

3 Place duck breasts skin side down in large skillet over medium heat; cook without turning 10 to 12 minutes or until skin is crisp and golden brown. Turn and cook about 8 minutes or until medium rare (130°F). Remove duck to plate; let stand 10 minutes before slicing.

4 Meanwhile, drain all but 1 tablespoon fat from skillet. Add shallot to skillet; cook and stir over medium heat 2 to 3 minutes or until translucent. Add vinegar mixture; cook and stir about 5 minutes or until slightly thickened. Season with salt and pepper. Slice duck; drizzle with sauce.

MAKES 4 SERVINGS

PER SERVING

CALORIES 360, TOTAL FAT 18g, CARBS 5g, NET CARBS 5g, DIETARY FIBER 0g, PROTEIN 42g

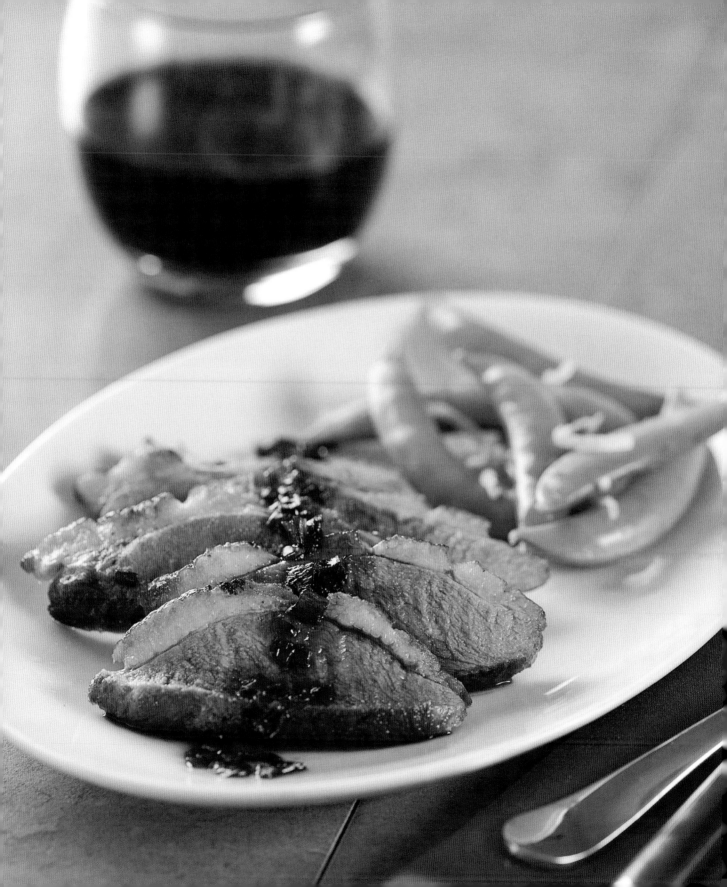

CHEESY CHICKEN AND BACON

½ cup Dijon mustard

4 tablespoons olive oil, divided

1 teaspoon lemon juice

4 boneless skinless chicken breasts (about 6 ounces each)

Salt and black pepper

1 tablespoon butter

2 cups sliced mushrooms

4 slices bacon, cooked

½ cup (2 ounces) shredded Cheddar cheese

½ cup (2 ounces) shredded Monterey Jack cheese

Chopped fresh parsley

1 Whisk mustard, 3 tablespoons oil and lemon juice in medium bowl until well blended. Remove half of marinade mixture to use as sauce; cover and refrigerate until ready to serve.

2 Place chicken in large resealable food storage bag. Pour remaining half of marinade over chicken; seal bag and turn to coat. Refrigerate at least 2 hours.

3 Preheat oven to 375°F. Remove chicken from marinade; discard marinade. Heat remaining 1 tablespoon oil in large ovenproof skillet over medium-high heat. Add chicken; cook 3 to 4 minutes per side or until golden brown. (Chicken will not be cooked through.) Remove chicken to plate; sprinkle with salt and pepper.

4 Heat butter in same skillet over medium-high heat. Add mushrooms; cook 8 minutes or until mushrooms begin to brown, stirring occasionally and scraping up browned bits from bottom of skillet. Season with salt and pepper. Return chicken to skillet; spoon mushrooms over chicken. Top with bacon; sprinkle with Cheddar and Monterey Jack cheeses.

5 Bake 8 to 10 minutes or until chicken is no longer pink in center and cheeses are melted. Sprinkle with parsley; serve with reserved mustard mixture.

MAKES 4 SERVINGS

PER SERVING

CALORIES 610, TOTAL FAT 41g, CARBS 2g, NET CARBS 2g, DIETARY FIBER 0g, PROTEIN 49g

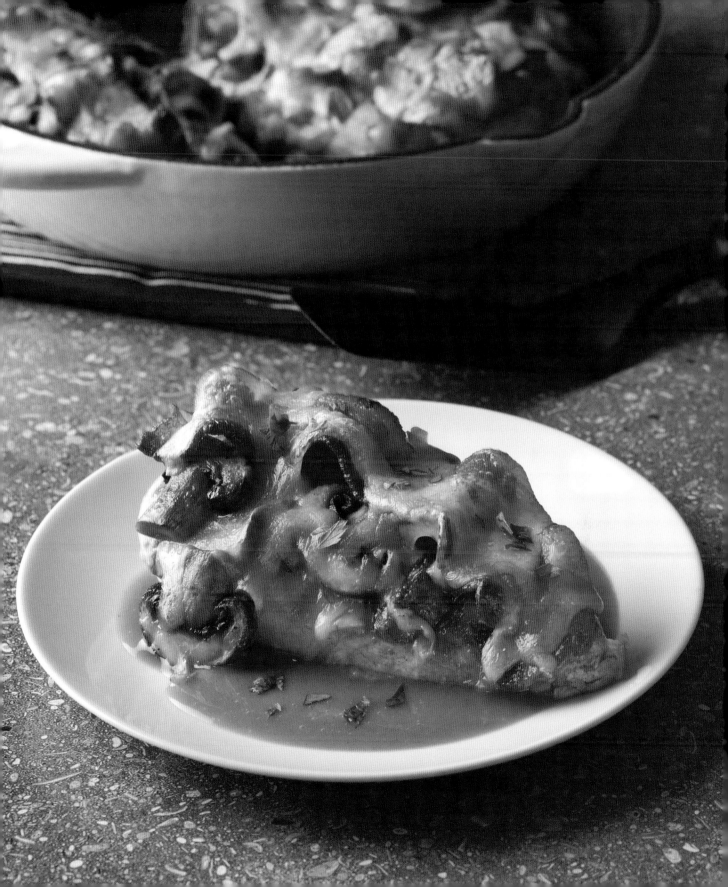

FORTY-CLOVE CHICKEN FILICE

¼ cup olive oil

1 cut-up whole chicken
(about 3 pounds)

40 cloves garlic (about
2 heads), peeled

4 stalks celery, thickly
sliced

½ cup dry white wine*

¼ cup dry vermouth*

Grated peel and
juice of 1 lemon

2 tablespoons finely
chopped fresh
parsley

2 teaspoons dried
basil

1 teaspoon dried
oregano, crushed

Pinch of red pepper
flakes

Salt and black
pepper

*Or substitute ¾ cup
chicken broth for the wine
and the vermouth.*

1 Preheat oven to 375°F.

2 Heat oil in Dutch oven. Add chicken; cook until browned
on all sides.

3 Add garlic, celery, wine, vermouth, lemon juice, parsley,
basil, oregano and red pepper flakes; mix well. Sprinkle
with lemon peel; season with salt and black pepper.

4 Cover and bake 40 minutes. Remove cover; bake
15 minutes or until chicken is cooked through (165°F).

MAKES 4 SERVINGS

PER SERVING

CALORIES 400, TOTAL FAT 22g, CARBS 13g,
NET CARBS 11g, DIETARY FIBER 2g, PROTEIN 34g

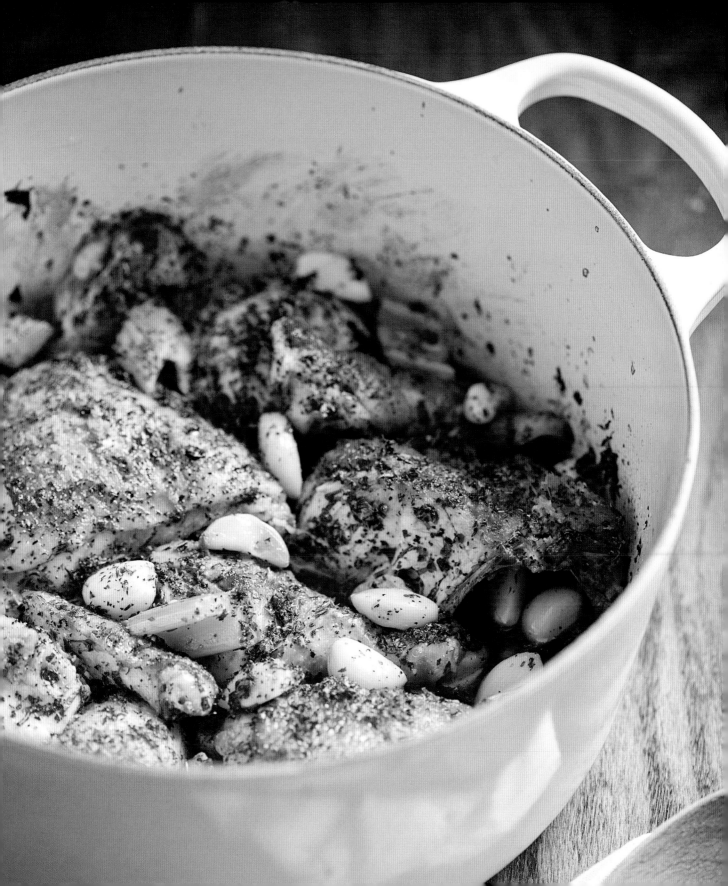

CILANTRO-STUFFED CHICKEN BREASTS

2 cloves garlic
1 cup packed fresh
    cilantro leaves
1 tablespoon plus
    2 teaspoons soy
    sauce, divided
1 tablespoon peanut
    or vegetable oil
4 boneless chicken
    breasts (about
    6 ounces each)
1 tablespoon dark
    sesame oil

1 Preheat oven to 350°F. Line sheet pan with foil; place wire rack on pan. Mince garlic in blender or food processor. Add cilantro; process until cilantro is minced. Add 2 teaspoons soy sauce and peanut oil; process until paste forms.

2 With rubber spatula or fingers, spread about 1 tablespoon cilantro mixture evenly under skin of each chicken breast, taking care not to puncture skin.

3 Place chicken on rack. Combine remaining 1 tablespoon soy sauce and sesame oil in small bowl. Brush half of mixture evenly over chicken. Bake 25 minutes; brush remaining soy sauce mixture evenly over chicken. Bake 10 minutes or until chicken is cooked through (165°F) and juices run clear.

MAKES 4 SERVINGS

PER SERVING

CALORIES 180, TOTAL FAT 9g, CARBS 1g, NET CARBS 1g, DIETARY FIBER 0g, PROTEIN 21g

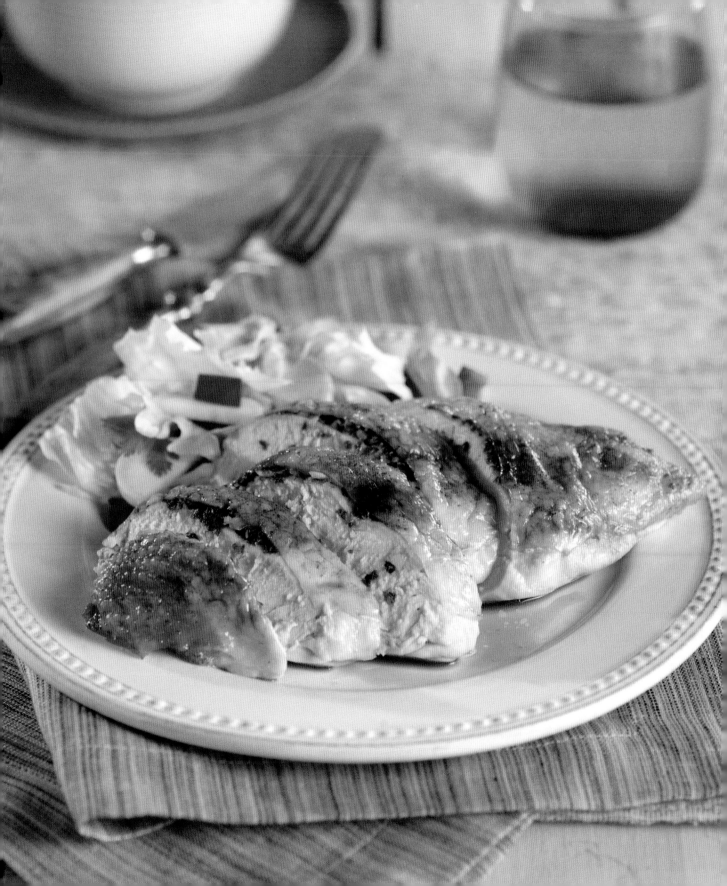

SWISS, TOMATO AND TURKEY PATTY MELT

1 pound ground turkey

½ packet (0.4 ounce) ranch salad dressing mix

1 medium green onion, finely chopped

1 teaspoon olive oil

2 slices Swiss cheese, halved diagonally

1 medium tomato, diced

1 Combine turkey, salad dressing mix and green onion in medium bowl; mix well. Shape into 4 patties.

2 Spray large nonstick skillet with nonstick cooking spray; heat over medium heat. Add oil; tilt skillet to coat bottom. Add patties. Cook 14 minutes or until cooked through (165°F), turning once.

3 Remove skillet from heat. Top each patty with cheese. Cover and let stand 2 to 3 minutes or until cheese is melted. Top each patty with tomatoes.

MAKES 4 SERVINGS

PER SERVING

CALORIES 239, TOTAL FAT 11g, CARBS 3g, NET CARBS 2g, DIETARY FIBER 1g, PROTEIN 28g

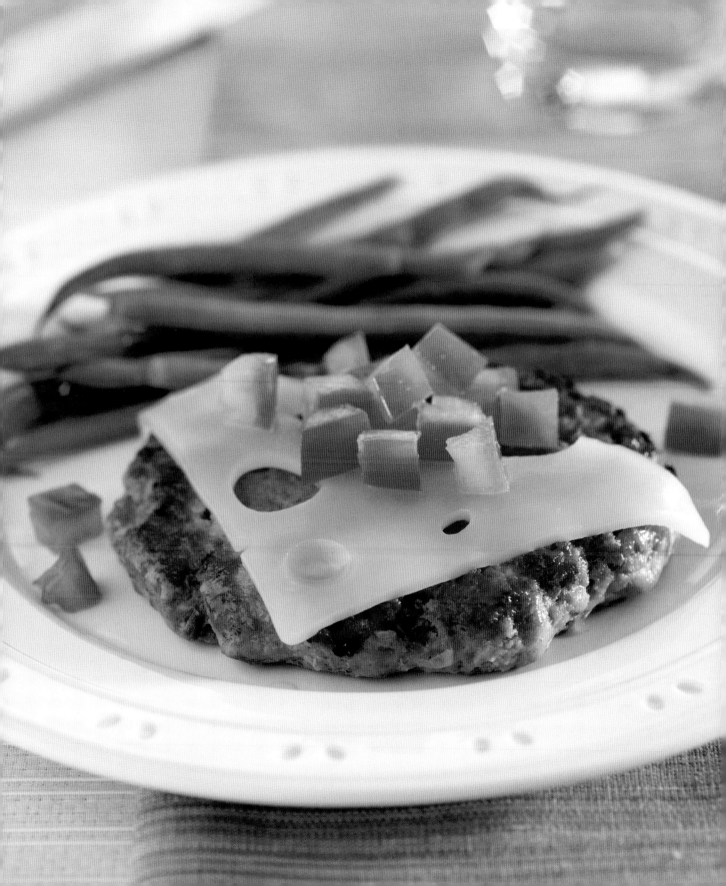

CHICKEN WITH ARTICHOKES

½ **teaspoon salt, divided**

⅛ **teaspoon black pepper**

4 **boneless skinless chicken breasts**

2 **tablespoons olive oil**

½ **medium red pepper, cut into thin strips**

2 **cloves garlic, minced**

1 **package (9 ounces) frozen artichoke hearts**

¾ **cup chicken broth**

1 **tablespoon lemon juice**

½ **teaspoon dried marjoram**

1 Sprinkle ¼ teaspoon salt and pepper over chicken. Heat oil in large skillet over medium-high heat. Add red pepper strips; cook and stir 2 to 3 minutes or until tender. Transfer to small bowl.

2 Add chicken; cook about 6 minutes, turning once, or until browned on both sides. Add garlic; cook 1 minute. Add artichoke hearts, broth, lemon juice, marjoram and remaining ¼ teaspoon salt. Bring to a boil. Reduce heat; cover and cook about 10 minutes or until chicken and artichokes are fork-tender. Top with red pepper strips.

MAKES 4 SERVINGS

PER SERVING

CALORIES 240, TOTAL FAT 11g, CARBS 8g, NET CARBS 3g, DIETARY FIBER 5g, PROTEIN 28g

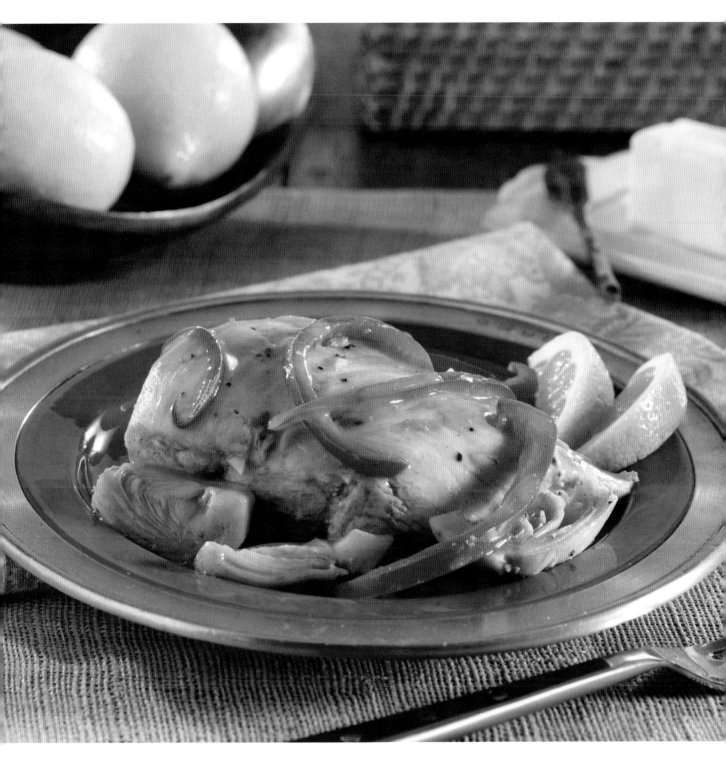

INDIAN-INSPIRED CHICKEN WITH RAITA

1 cup plain yogurt

2 cloves garlic, minced

1 teaspoon salt

1 teaspoon ground coriander

1 teaspoon ground ginger

½ teaspoon ground turmeric

½ teaspoon ground cinnamon

½ teaspoon ground cumin

¼ teaspoon ground red pepper

1 (5- to 6-pound) chicken, cut into 8 pieces (about 4 pounds chicken parts)

RAITA

2 medium cucumbers (about 1 pound), peeled, seeded and thinly sliced

⅓ cup plain yogurt

2 tablespoons chopped fresh cilantro

1 clove garlic, minced

¼ teaspoon salt

⅛ teaspoon black pepper

1 Mix 1 cup yogurt, 2 cloves garlic, 1 teaspoon salt, coriander, ginger, turmeric, cinnamon, cumin and red pepper in medium bowl. Place chicken in large resealable food storage bag. Add yogurt mixture. Seal bag; turn to coat. Marinate in refrigerator 4 to 24 hours, turning occasionally.

2 Preheat broiler. Cover baking sheet with foil. Place chicken on prepared baking sheet; discard marinade. Broil 6 inches from heat source about 30 minutes or until cooked through (165°F), turning once.

3 Meanwhile for raita, combine cucumbers, ⅓ cup yogurt, cilantro, 1 clove garlic, ¼ teaspoon salt and black pepper in small bowl. Serve with chicken.

MAKES 6 SERVINGS

PER SERVING

CALORIES 625, TOTAL FAT 43g, CARBS 8g, NET CARBS 7g, DIETARY FIBER 1g, PROTEIN 50g

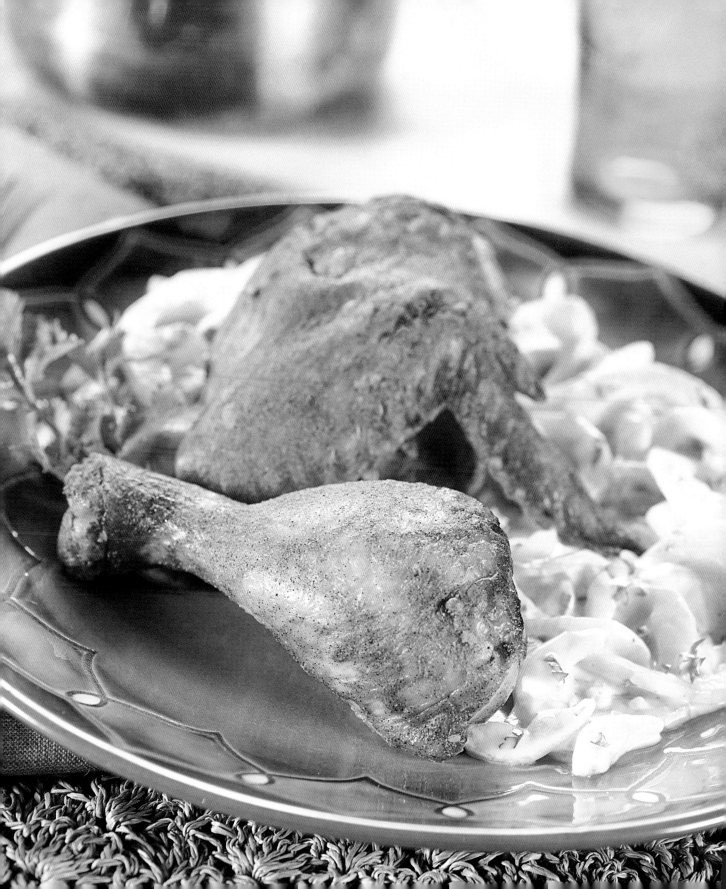

SWEET SPICED TARRAGON ROAST TURKEY BREAST

2 tablespoons canola or corn oil

2 teaspoons grated orange peel

1½ teaspoons dried tarragon

1 teaspoon ground cumin

½ teaspoon ground allspice

½ teaspoon ground cinnamon

½ teaspoon ground ginger

½ teaspoon salt

½ teaspoon black pepper

¼ teaspoon ground red pepper

1 (2½-pound) turkey breast half (with bone in), thawed

1 Preheat oven to 400°F. Whisk oil, orange peel, tarragon, cumin, allspice, cinnamon, ginger, salt, black pepper and red pepper in small bowl. Loosen skin from turkey and gently rub spice mixture under skin.

2 Spray broiler pan with nonstick cooking spray. Place turkey, skin side up, on prepared pan. Bake 1 hour 15 minutes or until meat reaches 165°F when tested with instant-read thermometer. Let stand 15 minutes. Remove and discard skin, leaving spice mixture on turkey. Thinly slice turkey.

MAKES 6 SERVINGS

PER SERVING

CALORIES 220, TOTAL FAT 7g, CARBS 1g, NET CARBS 1g, DIETARY FIBER 0g, PROTEIN 36g

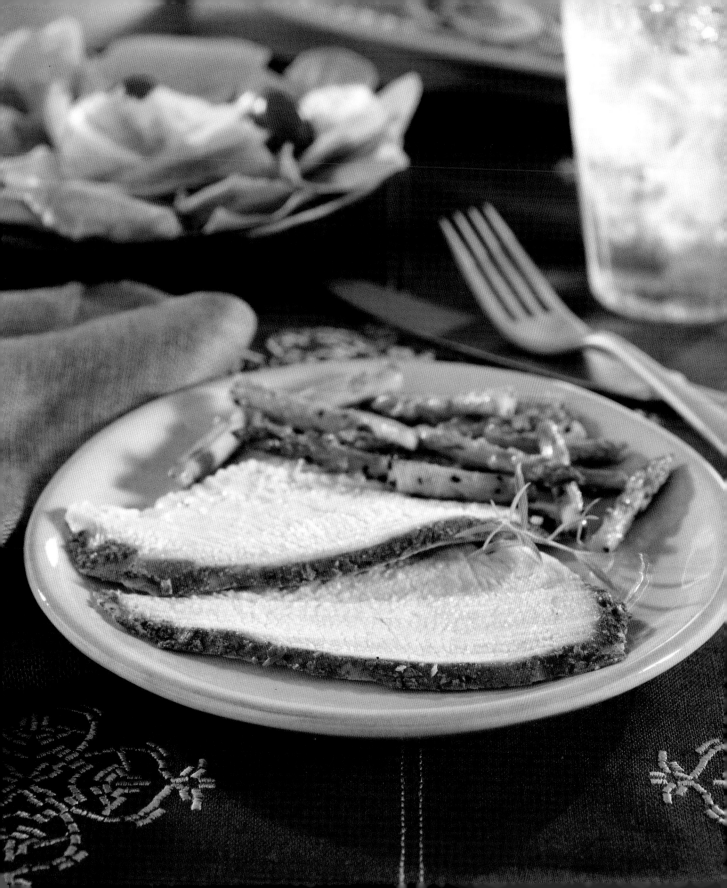

GREEK LEMON CHICKEN

4 boneless skinless chicken breasts (about 4 ounces each)

2 tablespoons lemon juice

2 teaspoons extra virgin olive oil

1 teaspoon grated lemon peel

1 teaspoon dried oregano

1 clove garlic, minced

¼ teaspoon salt

⅛ teaspoon black pepper

1 lemon, cut into wedges (optional)

1 Place chicken in large resealable food storage bag. Add lemon juice, oil, lemon peel, oregano, garlic, salt and pepper. Seal bag; shake to coat chicken. Marinate in refrigerator at least 30 minutes or up to 8 hours.

2 Spray large nonstick skillet with nonstick cooking spray; heat over medium heat. Remove chicken from marinade; discard marinade. Add chicken to skillet; cook 3 minutes. Turn chicken. Reduce heat to medium-low. Cook about 7 minutes or until no longer pink in center.

3 Remove from heat. Serve with lemon wedges, if desired.

MAKES 4 SERVINGS

PER SERVING

CALORIES 132, TOTAL FAT 2g, CARBS 3g, NET CARBS 2g, DIETARY FIBER 1g, PROTEIN 27g

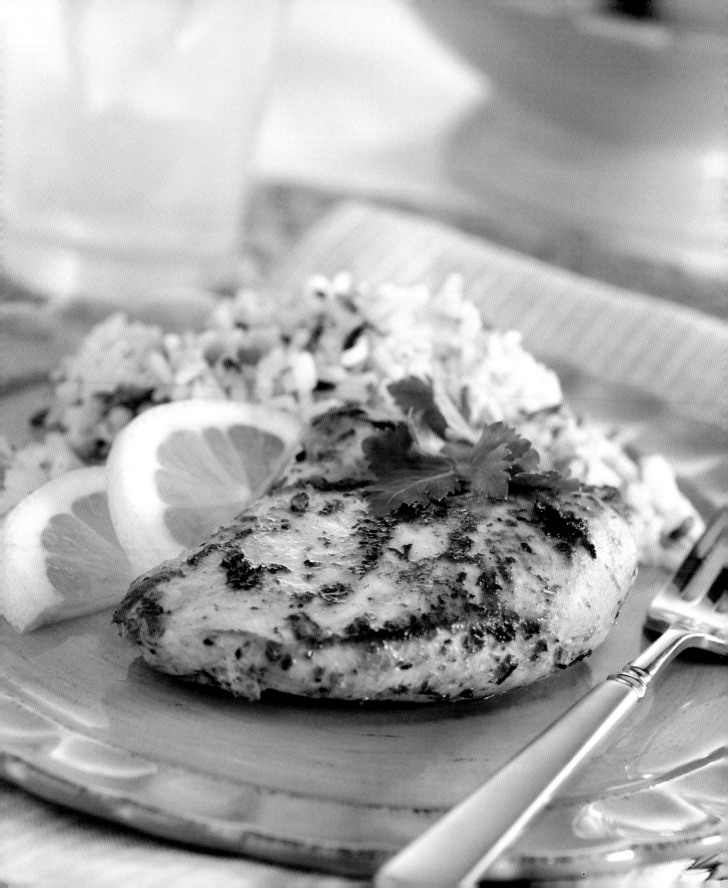

QUICK AND EASY SAUTÉED CHICKEN

4 boneless skinless
  chicken breasts
  (4 ounces each)
1 teaspoon smoked or
  sweet paprika
1 teaspoon dried
  thyme
½ teaspoon garlic salt
⅛ teaspoon ground red
  pepper
2 teaspoons olive oil

1 Place chicken breasts between sheets of waxed paper or plastic wrap; pound to even ½-inch thickness. Combine paprika, thyme, garlic salt and red pepper in small bowl; rub over both sides of chicken.

2 Heat oil in large nonstick skillet over medium heat. Add chicken; cook 4 to 5 minutes per side or until chicken is no longer pink in center. Pour any juices from skillet over chicken.

MAKES 4 SERVINGS

PER SERVING

CALORIES 147, TOTAL FAT 4g, CARBS 1g, NET CARBS 0g, DIETARY FIBER 1g, PROTEIN 26g

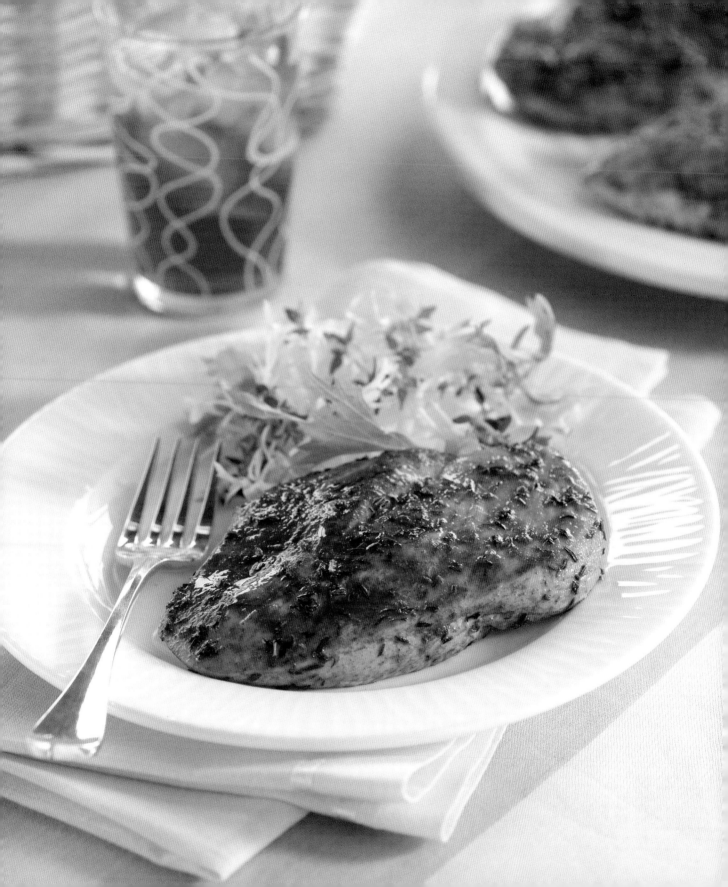

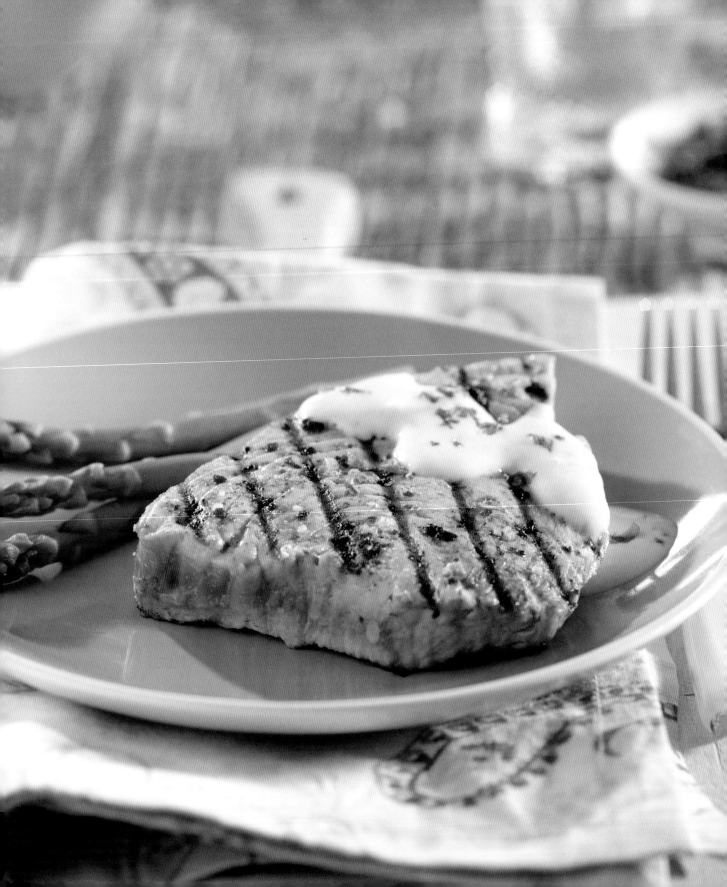

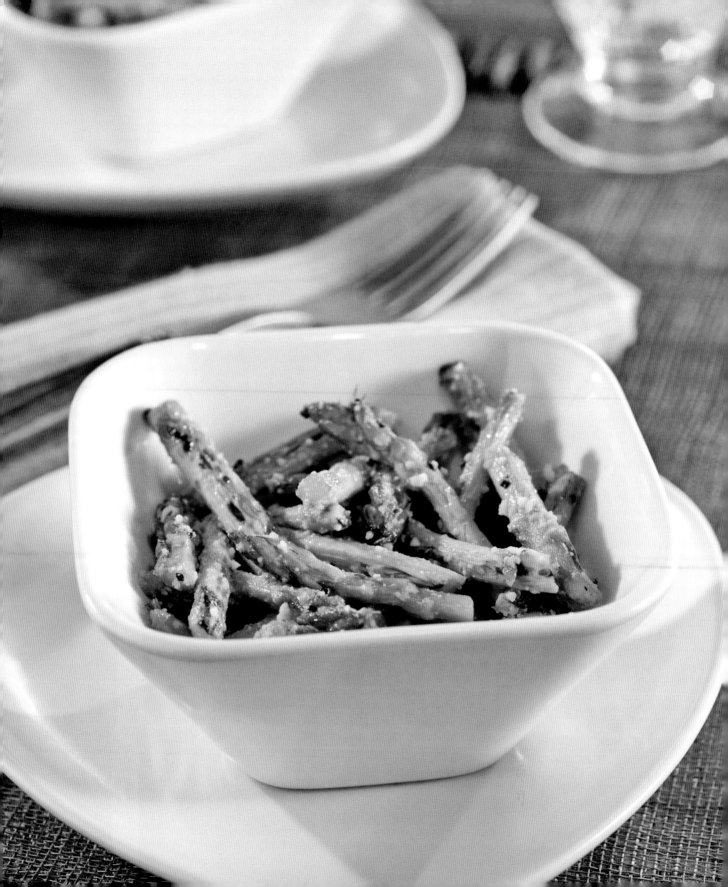

SAUTÉED KALE WITH MUSHROOMS AND BACON

1 slice uncooked bacon, chopped

½ cup sliced shallots

1 package (4 ounces) sliced mixed exotic mushrooms *or* 8 ounces cremini mushrooms, sliced

10 cups loosely packed torn fresh kale leaves (about 8 ounces),* stems removed

2 tablespoons water

½ teaspoon black pepper

Buy loose kale leaves or look for 16-ounce bags of ready-to-cook fresh kale leaves in the produce section of the supermarket.

1 Cook bacon in large heavy skillet over medium heat 5 minutes. Add shallots; cook and stir 3 minutes. Add mushrooms; cook and stir 8 minutes.

2 Add kale and water; cover and cook 5 minutes. Uncover; cook and stir 5 minutes or until kale is crisp-tender. Season with pepper.

MAKES 4 SERVINGS

PER SERVING

CALORIES 90, TOTAL FAT 4g, CARBS 11g, NET CARBS 8g, DIETARY FIBER 3g, PROTEIN 4g

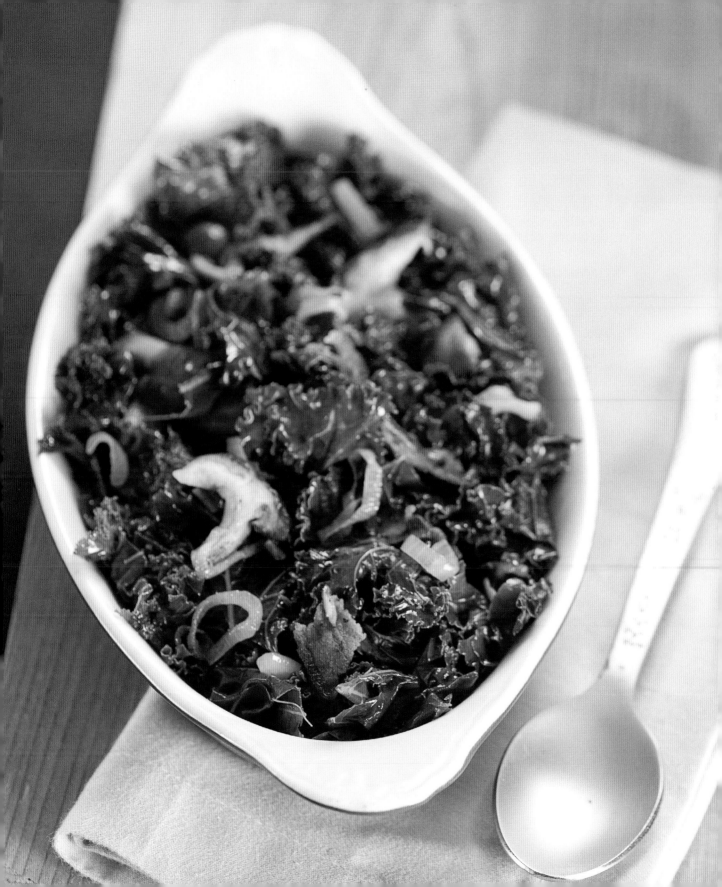

BACON AND CHEESE DIP

2 packages (8 ounces each) cream cheese, cut into cubes

4 cups (16 ounces) shredded Colby-Jack cheese

1 cup half-and-half

2 tablespoons prepared mustard

1 tablespoon minced onion

2 teaspoons Worcestershire sauce

½ teaspoon salt

¼ teaspoon hot pepper sauce

1 pound bacon, crisp-cooked and crumbled

Cut-up fresh vegetables

SLOW COOKER DIRECTIONS

1 Combine cream cheese, Colby-Jack cheese, half-and-half, mustard, onion, Worcestershire sauce, salt and pepper sauce in 1½-quart slow cooker.

2 Cover; cook on LOW 1 hour or until cheese melts, stirring occasionally.

3 Stir in bacon; adjust seasonings. Serve with vegetables.

MAKES ABOUT 16 SERVINGS (4 TABLESPOONS EACH)

PER SERVING

CALORIES 360, TOTAL FAT 29g, CARBS 3g, NET CARBS 3g, DIETARY FIBER 0g, PROTEIN 20g

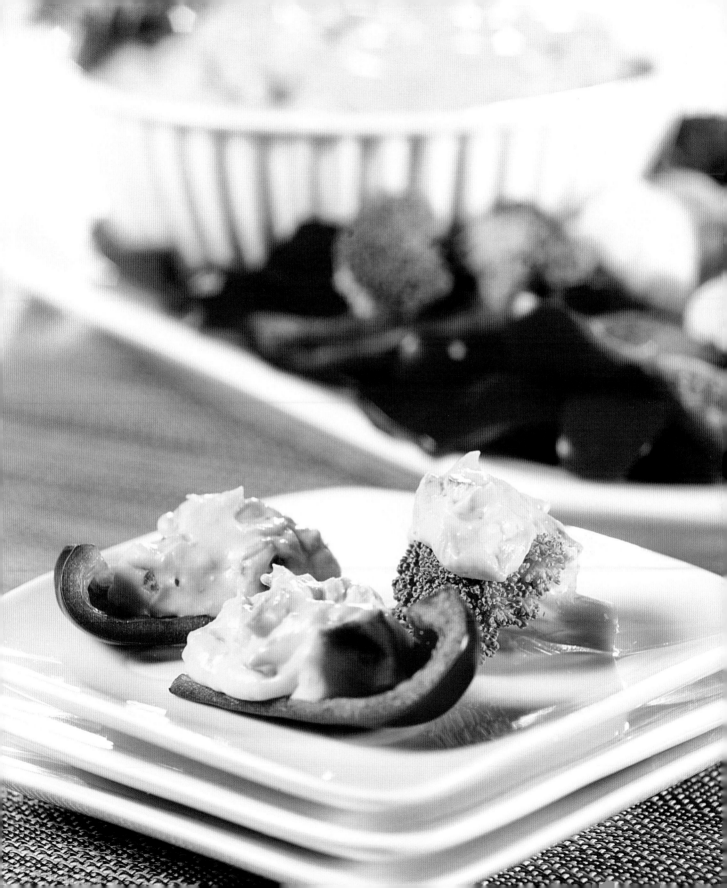

ZUCCHINI WITH FETA CASSEROLE

4 medium zucchini

1 tablespoon butter

2 eggs, beaten

½ cup grated Parmesan cheese

⅓ cup crumbled feta cheese

2 tablespoons chopped fresh parsley

2 teaspoons chopped fresh marjoram

Dash hot pepper sauce

Salt and black pepper

1 Preheat oven to 375°F. Spray 2-quart casserole with nonstick cooking spray.

2 Grate zucchini; drain in colander. Melt butter in large skillet over medium heat. Add zucchini; cook and stir until slightly browned.

3 Remove from heat; stir in eggs, cheeses, parsley, marjoram, hot pepper sauce, salt and black pepper until well blended. Pour into prepared casserole.

4 Bake 35 minutes or until hot and bubbly.

MAKES 4 SERVINGS

PER SERVING

CALORIES 220, TOTAL FAT 14g, CARBS 12g, NET CARBS 9g, DIETARY FIBER 3g, PROTEIN 15g

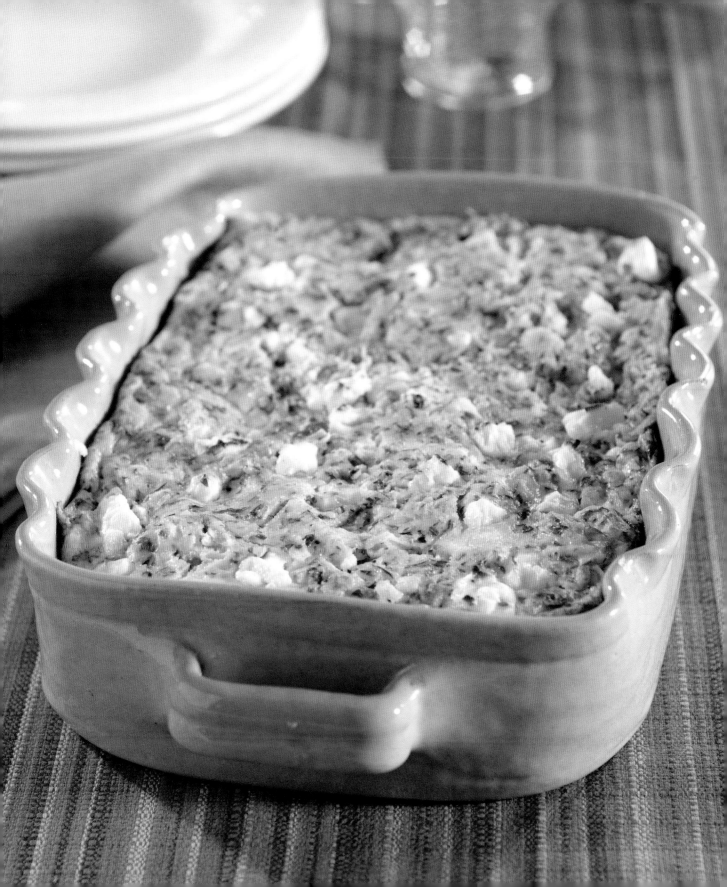

AVOCADO SALSA

1 medium avocado, diced

1 cup chopped onion

1 cup peeled seeded chopped cucumber

1 Anaheim pepper, seeded and chopped

½ cup chopped fresh tomato

2 tablespoons chopped fresh cilantro

½ teaspoon salt

¼ teaspoon hot pepper sauce

1 Combine avocado, onion, cucumber, Anaheim pepper, tomato, salt and hot pepper sauce in medium bowl; mix gently.

2 Cover and refrigerate at least 1 hour before serving.

MAKES 32 SERVINGS (2 TABLESPOONS EACH)

PER SERVING

CALORIES 13, TOTAL FAT 1g, CARBS 1g, NET CARBS 0g, DIETARY FIBER 1g, PROTEIN 1g

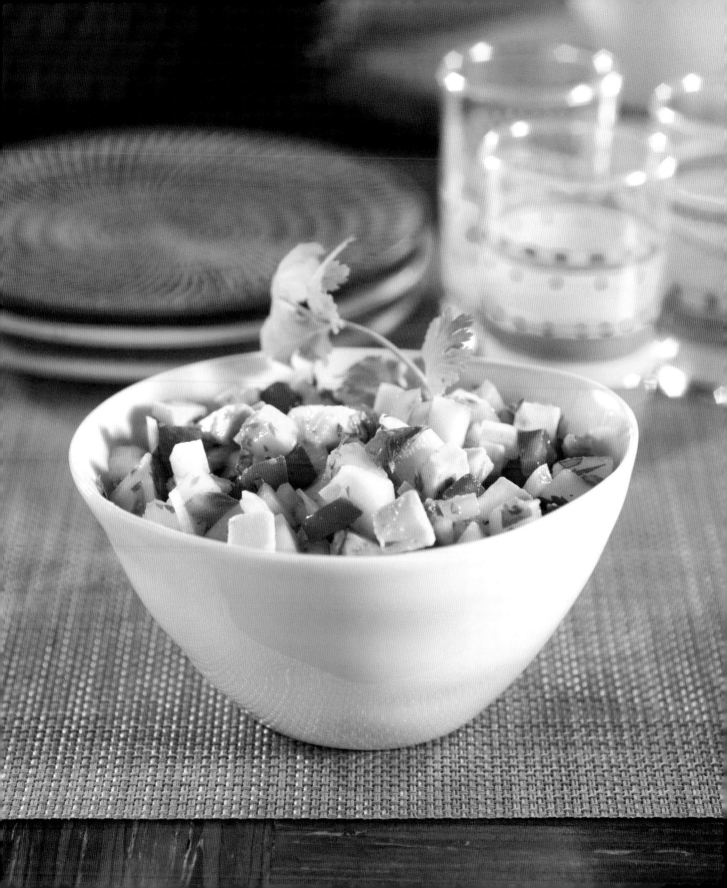

DILLED BRUSSELS SPROUTS

1 package (10 ounces) frozen brussels sprouts *or* 1 pint fresh brussels sprouts

½ cup beef broth

1 teaspoon dill seed

1 teaspoon dried minced onion

Salt and black pepper

1 Combine brussels sprouts, broth, dill and onion in medium saucepan. Bring to a simmer over medium heat. Reduce heat to medium-low; cover and simmer 8 to 10 minutes or until sprouts are nearly tender.

2 Uncover and continue to simmer until most of liquid is evaporated. Season with salt and black pepper.

MAKES 3 SERVINGS

PER SERVING

CALORIES 43, TOTAL FAT 1g, CARBS 8g, NET CARBS 5g, DIETARY FIBER 3g, PROTEIN 4g

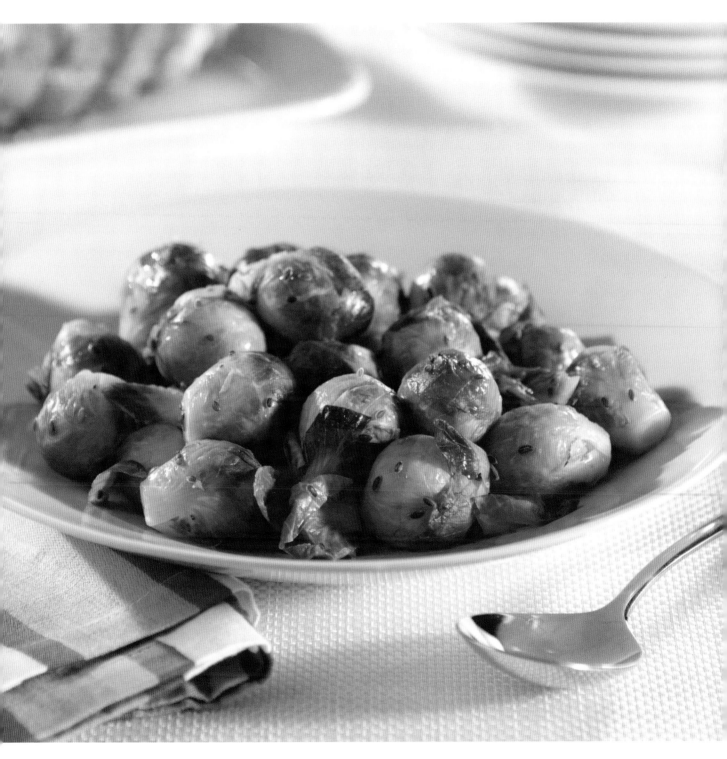

PICANTE VEGETABLE DIP

⅔ cup reduced-fat sour cream

½ cup picante sauce

⅓ cup mayonnaise

¼ cup finely chopped green or red bell pepper

2 tablespoons finely chopped green onion

¾ teaspoon garlic salt

Cut-up fresh vegetables

1 Combine sour cream, picante sauce, mayonnaise, bell pepper, green onion and garlic salt in medium bowl until well blended.

2 Cover; refrigerate several hours or overnight to allow flavors to blend. Serve with vegetables.

MAKES 13 SERVINGS (2 TABLESPOONS EACH)

PER SERVING

CALORIES 61, TOTAL FAT 6g, CARBS 2g, NET CARBS 1g, DIETARY FIBER 1g, PROTEIN 1g

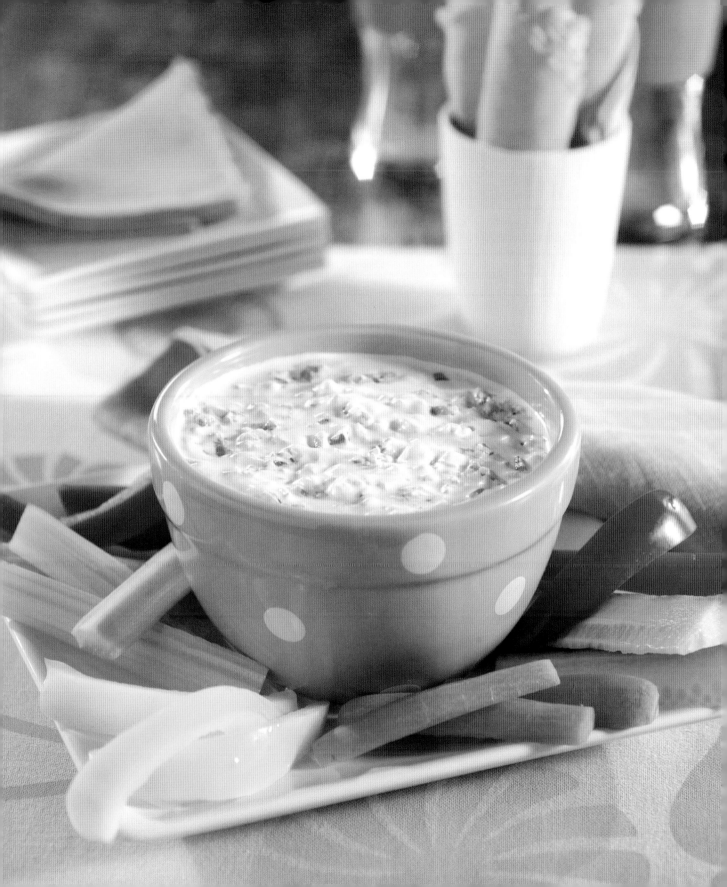

BROCCOLI AND CHEESE

2 medium crowns broccoli (1½ pounds), cut into florets (about 6½ cups)

2 tablespoons butter

1½ cups milk

½ teaspoon salt

⅛ teaspoon ground nutmeg

⅛ teaspoon ground red pepper

1 cup (4 ounces) shredded Cheddar cheese

½ cup (2 ounces) shredded Monterey Jack cheese

¼ cup shredded Parmesan cheese

Paprika (optional)

1 Bring large saucepan of water to a boil over medium-high heat. Add broccoli; cook 7 minutes or until tender. Drain and place in serving bowl; keep warm.

2 Melt butter in same saucepan over medium heat. Stir in milk; bring to a simmer, whisking frequently. Simmer 5 minutes, whisking constantly. Stir in salt, nutmeg and red pepper. Reduce heat to low; whisk in cheeses in three additions, whisking well after first two additions and stirring just until blended after last addition.

3 Pour sauce over broccoli; sprinkle with paprika. Serve immediately.

MAKES 4 SERVINGS

PER SERVING

CALORIES 340, TOTAL FAT 24g, CARBS 14g, NET CARBS 10g, DIETARY FIBER 4g, PROTEIN 19g

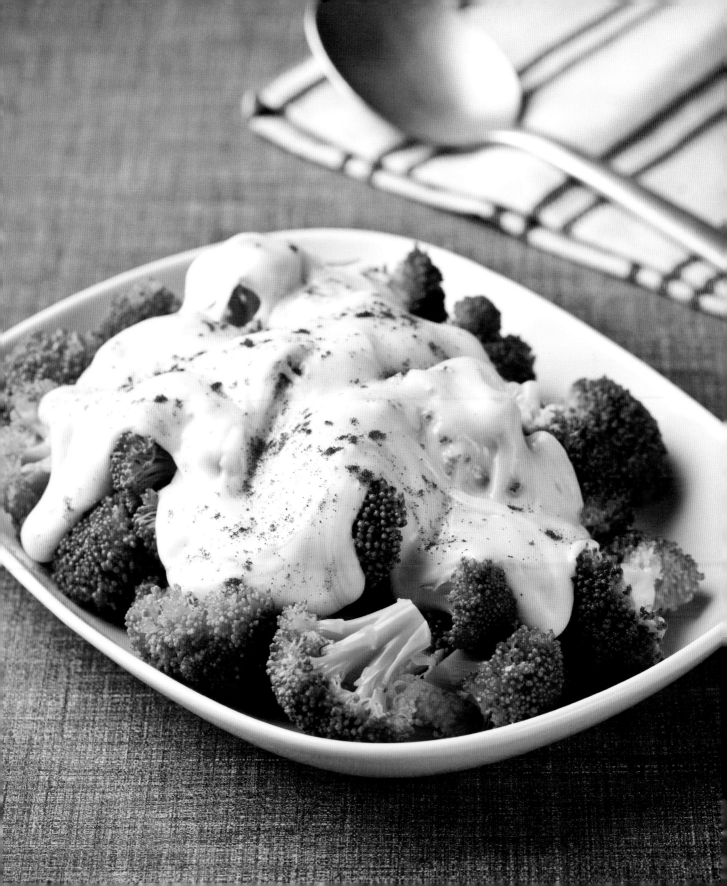

BUFFALO CHICKEN DIP

2 packages (8 ounces each) cream cheese, softened and cut into pieces

1 jar (12 ounces) restaurant-style wing sauce

1 cup ranch dressing

2 cups shredded cooked chicken (from 1 pound boneless skinless chicken breasts)

2 cups (8 ounces) shredded Cheddar cheese

Celery sticks

1 Combine cream cheese, wing sauce and ranch dressing in large saucepan; cook over medium-low heat 7 to 10 minutes or until cream cheese is melted and mixture is smooth, whisking frequently.

2 Combine chicken and Cheddar cheese in large bowl. Add cream cheese mixture; stir until well blended. Pour into serving bowl; serve warm with celery sticks.

MAKES 20 SERVINGS (4 TABLESPOONS EACH)

PER SERVING

CALORIES 190, TOTAL FAT 15g, CARBS 3g, NET CARBS 3g, DIETARY FIBER 0g, PROTEIN 9g

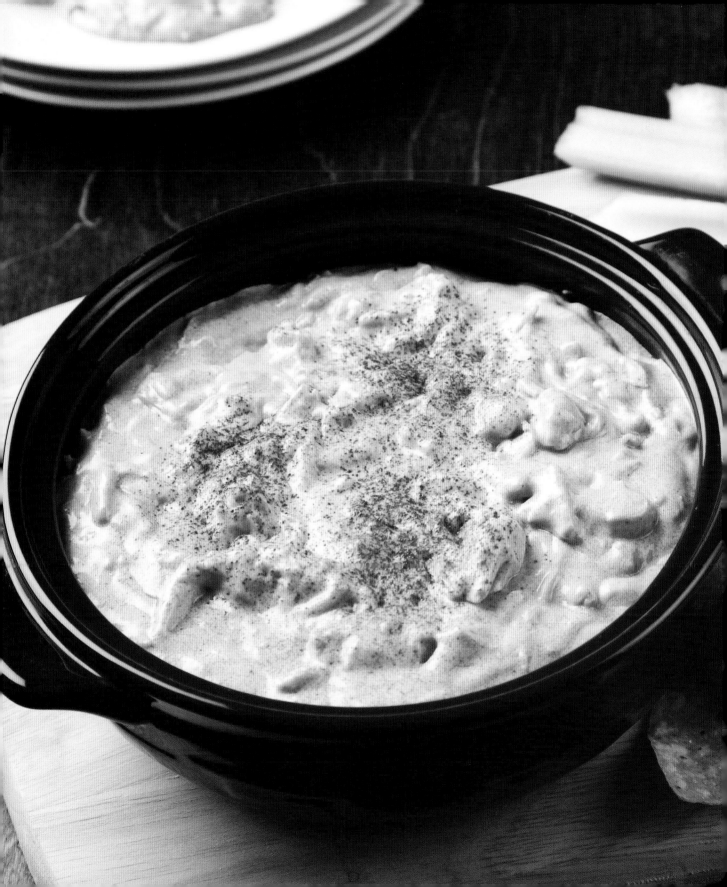

BRUSSELS SPROUTS WITH BACON AND BUTTER

6 slices thick-cut bacon, cut into ½-inch pieces

1½ pounds brussels sprouts (about 24 medium), halved

¼ teaspoon salt

¼ teaspoon black pepper

2 tablespoons butter, softened

1 Preheat oven to 375°F. Cook bacon in large cast iron skillet until almost crisp. Drain on paper towel-lined plate; set aside. Drain all but 1 tablespoon drippings.

2 Add brussels sprouts to skillet. Sprinkle with ¼ teaspoon salt and ¼ teaspoon pepper; toss to coat. Spread in skillet.

3 Roast 30 minutes or until brussels sprouts are browned and crispy, stirring every 10 minutes.

4 Add butter to skillet; stir until completely coated. Stir in bacon; season with additional salt and pepper.

MAKES 4 SERVINGS

PER SERVING

CALORIES 220, TOTAL FAT 15g, CARBS 15g, NET CARBS 8g, DIETARY FIBER 7g, PROTEIN 10g

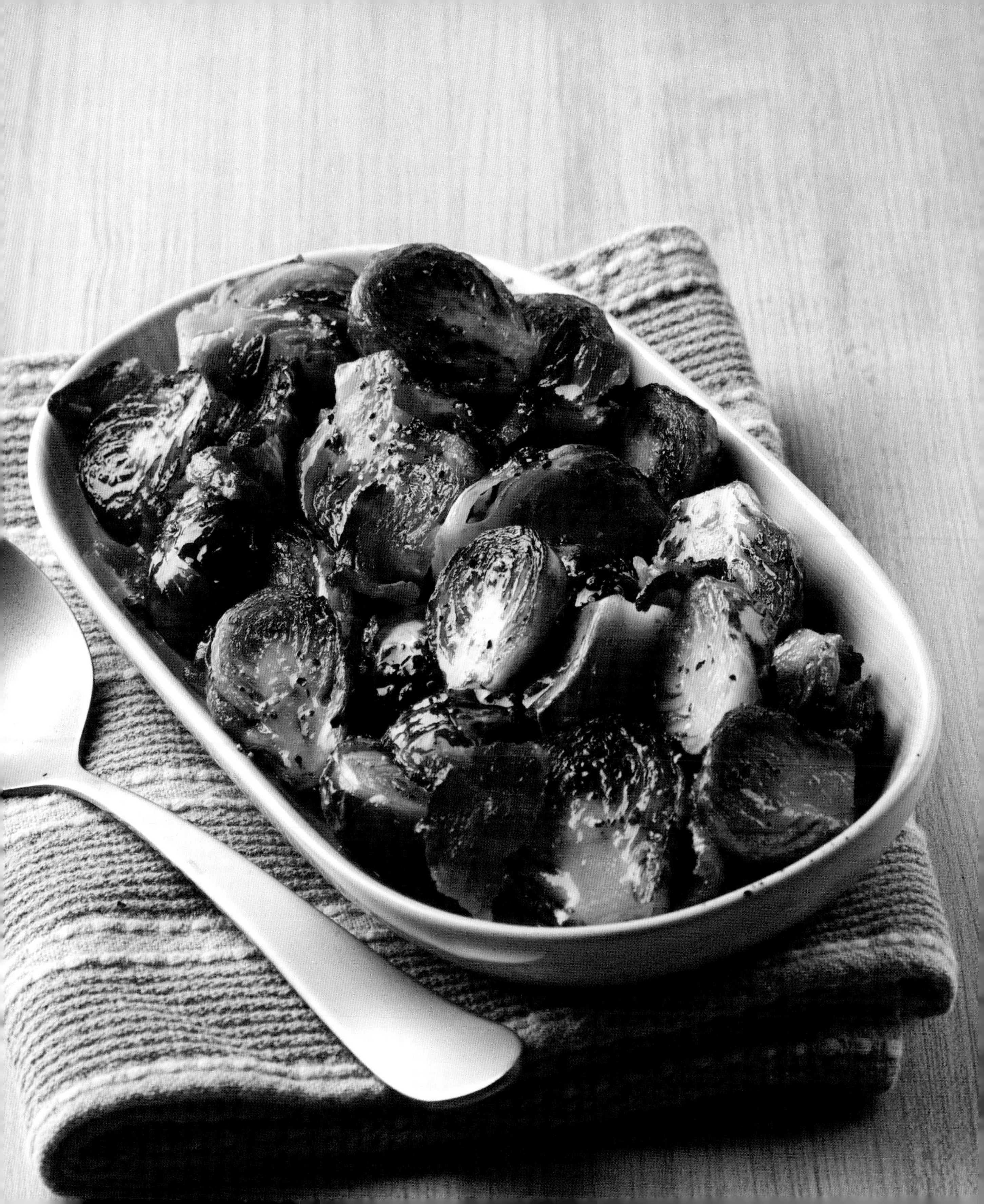

HERBED ZUCCHINI RIBBONS

2 tablespoons olive oil

1 tablespoon white wine vinegar

2 teaspoons chopped fresh basil *or* ½ teaspoon dried basil

½ teaspoon red pepper flakes

¼ teaspoon ground coriander

3 small zucchini (about 12 ounces total)

Salt and black pepper

1 Combine oil, vinegar, basil, red pepper flakes and coriander in large bowl; whisk until blended.

2 Cut tip and stem ends from zucchini with paring knife. Using vegetable peeler, begin at stem end and make continuous ribbons down length of each zucchini.

3 Place steamer basket in large saucepan; add 1 inch of water. (Water should not touch bottom of basket.) Place zucchini ribbons in steamer basket; cover. Bring to a boil over high heat. When pan begins to steam, check zucchini for doneness. (It should be crisp-tender.)

4 Transfer zucchini to bowl with dressing using slotted spatula or tongs; toss gently to coat. Season with salt and black pepper. Serve immediately or refrigerate up to 2 days.

MAKES 4 SERVINGS

PER SERVING

CALORIES 80, TOTAL FAT 7g, CARBS 3g, NET CARBS 2g, DIETARY FIBER 1g, PROTEIN 1g

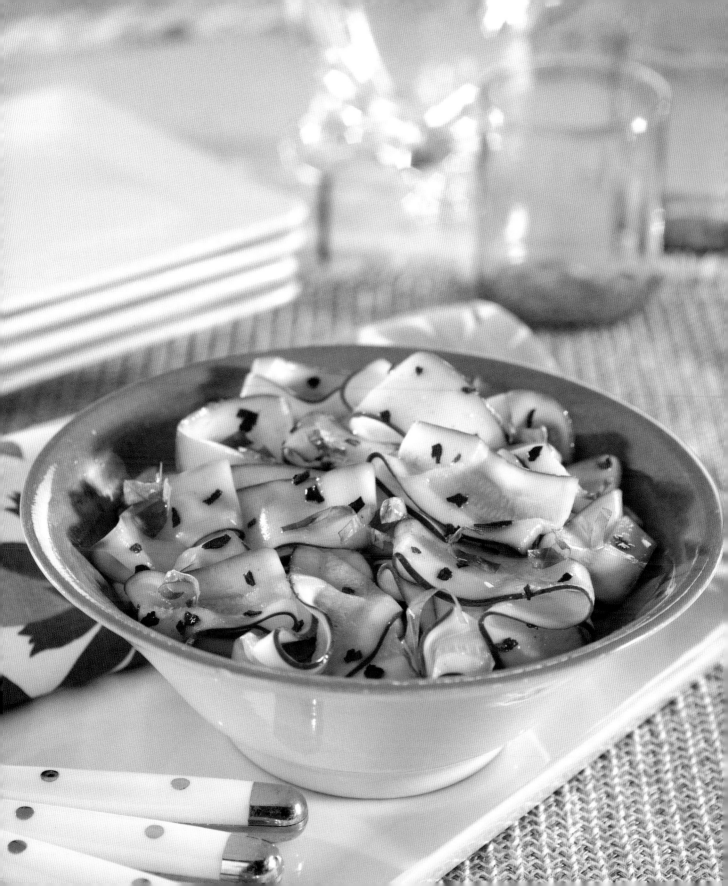

AVOCADO SMASH

1 ripe medium
   avocado

1 tablespoon lime
   juice

¼ cup plain nonfat
   Greek yogurt

1 teaspoon Dijon
   mustard

¼ teaspoon salt

Chopped fresh
   chives (optional)

Mash avocado with fork in shallow bowl to desired consistency. Stir in lime juice, yogurt, mustard and salt. Sprinkle with chives, if desired. Serve immediately.

MAKES 4 SERVINGS (3 TABLESPOONS EACH)

TIP

This dip is great with raw veggies, such as cucumber slices, celery sticks or red bell pepper strips.

PER SERVING

CALORIES 64, TOTAL FAT 5g, CARBS 4g, NET CARBS 2g, DIETARY FIBER 2g, PROTEIN 2g

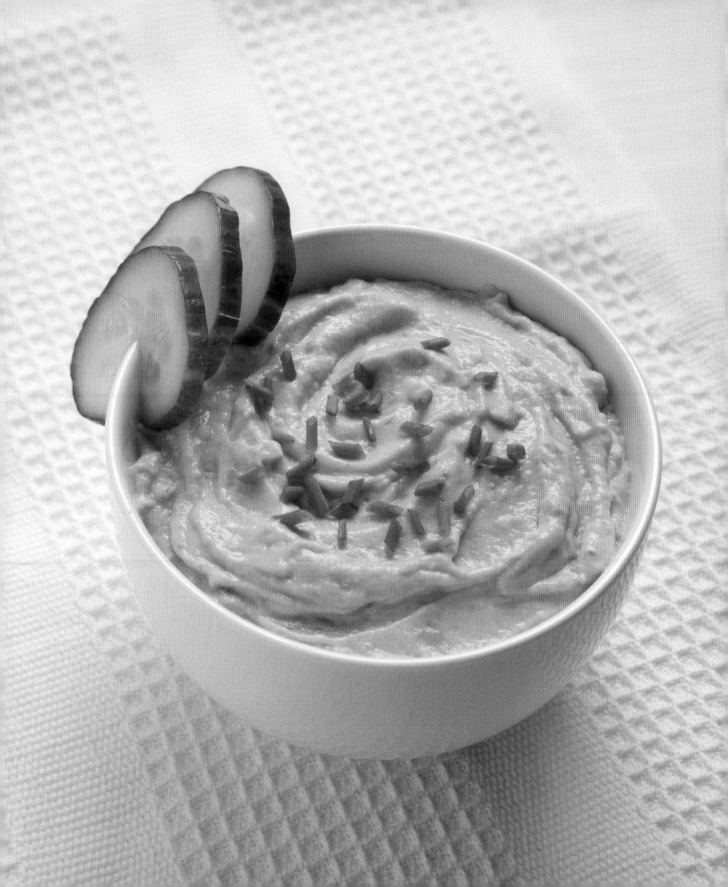

SMOKY KALE CHIFFONADE

12 ounces fresh young kale or mustard greens

3 slices bacon

2 tablespoons crumbled blue cheese

1 Rinse kale well in large bowl of warm water; drain in colander. Discard any discolored leaves; trim away tough stem ends. To prepare chiffonade, stack leaves and roll up into cylinder. Slice crosswise into ½-inch slices; separate into strips. Set aside.

2 Cook bacon in medium skillet over medium heat until crisp. Remove bacon to paper towel. Drain all but 1 tablespoon drippings.

3 Add kale to drippings in skillet. Cook and stir over medium-high heat 2 to 3 minutes until wilted and tender (older leaves may take slightly longer).

4 Crumble bacon. Toss bacon and blue cheese with kale. Serve immediately.

MAKES 4 SERVINGS

NOTE

"Chiffonade" in French literally means "made of rags." In cooking, it means "cut into thin strips."

PER SERVING

CALORIES 66, TOTAL FAT 4g, CARBS 5g, NET CARBS 4g, DIETARY FIBER 1g, PROTEIN 4g

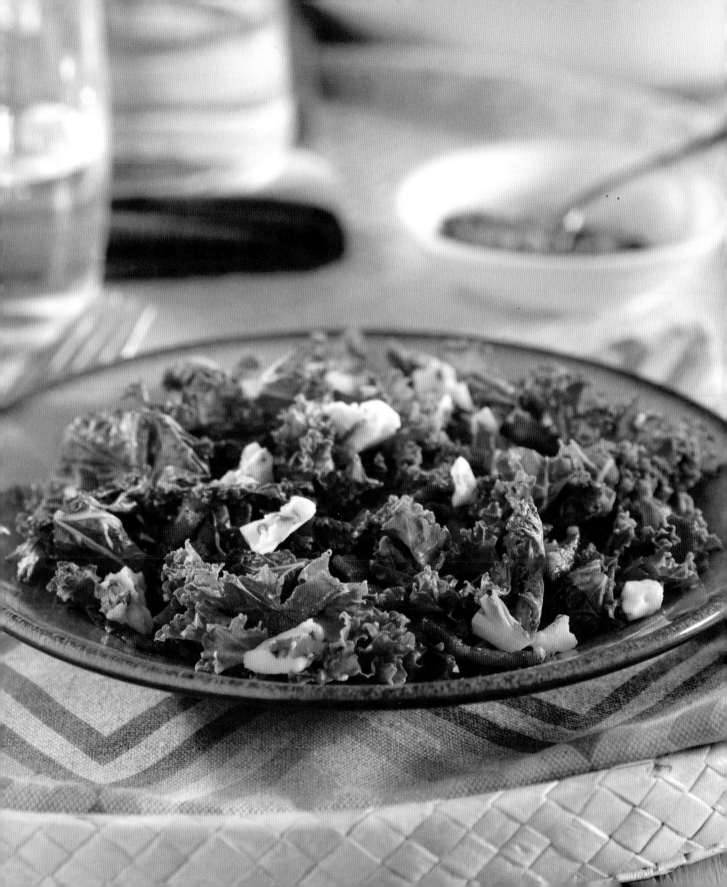

INDEX

INDEX

METRIC CONVERSION CHART

VOLUME MEASUREMENTS (dry)

$^1/_8$ teaspoon = 0.5 mL
$^1/_4$ teaspoon = 1 mL
$^1/_2$ teaspoon = 2 mL
$^3/_4$ teaspoon = 4 mL
1 teaspoon = 5 mL
1 tablespoon = 15 mL
2 tablespoons = 30 mL
$^1/_4$ cup = 60 mL
$^1/_3$ cup = 75 mL
$^1/_2$ cup = 125 mL
$^2/_3$ cup = 150 mL
$^3/_4$ cup = 175 mL
1 cup = 250 mL
2 cups = 1 pint = 500 mL
3 cups = 750 mL
4 cups = 1 quart = 1 L

VOLUME MEASUREMENTS (fluid)

1 fluid ounce (2 tablespoons) = 30 mL
4 fluid ounces ($^1/_2$ cup) = 125 mL
8 fluid ounces (1 cup) = 250 mL
12 fluid ounces ($1^1/_2$ cups) = 375 mL
16 fluid ounces (2 cups) = 500 mL

WEIGHTS (mass)

$^1/_2$ ounce = 15 g
1 ounce = 30 g
3 ounces = 90 g
4 ounces = 120 g
8 ounces = 225 g
10 ounces = 285 g
12 ounces = 360 g
16 ounces = 1 pound = 450 g

DIMENSIONS

$^1/_{16}$ inch = 2 mm
$^1/_8$ inch = 3 mm
$^1/_4$ inch = 6 mm
$^1/_2$ inch = 1.5 cm
$^3/_4$ inch = 2 cm
1 inch = 2.5 cm

OVEN TEMPERATURES

250°F = 120°C
275°F = 140°C
300°F = 150°C
325°F = 160°C
350°F = 180°C
375°F = 190°C
400°F = 200°C
425°F = 220°C
450°F = 230°C

BAKING PAN SIZES

Utensil	Size in Inches/Quarts	Metric Volume	Size in Centimeters
Baking or Cake Pan (square or rectangular)	8×8×2	2 L	20×20×5
	9×9×2	2.5 L	23×23×5
	12×8×2	3 L	30×20×5
	13×9×2	3.5 L	33×23×5
Loaf Pan	8×4×3	1.5 L	20×10×7
	9×5×3	2 L	23×13×7
Round Layer Cake Pan	8×1½	1.2 L	20×4
	9×1½	1.5 L	23×4
Pie Plate	8×1¼	750 mL	20×3
	9×1¼	1 L	23×3
Baking Dish or Casserole	1 quart	1 L	—
	1½ quart	1.5 L	—
	2 quart	2 L	—